T0329344

THE

GLOBAL CHALLENGE
OF MALARIA

Past Lessons and Future Prospects

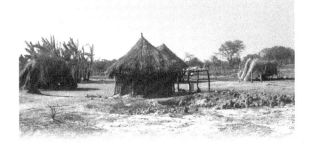

THE
GLOBAL CHALLENGE
OF MALARIA

Past Lessons and Future Prospects

Editors

Frank M Snowden • Richard Bucala
Yale University, USA

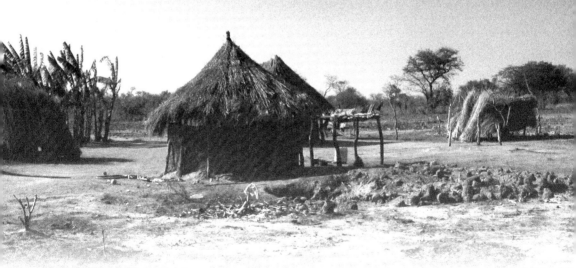

World Scientific

NEW JERSEY · LONDON · SINGAPORE · BEIJING · SHANGHAI · HONG KONG · TAIPEI · CHENNAI

Published by

World Scientific Publishing Co. Pte. Ltd.

5 Toh Tuck Link, Singapore 596224

USA office: 27 Warren Street, Suite 401-402, Hackensack, NJ 07601

UK office: 57 Shelton Street, Covent Garden, London WC2H 9HE

Library of Congress Cataloging-in-Publication Data
The global challenge of malaria : past lessons and future prospects / [edited by] Frank M. Snowden,
Richard Bucala.
    p. ; cm.
  ISBN 978-9814405577 (hardcover : alk. paper)
  I. Snowden, Frank M. (Frank Martin), 1946– editor of compilation. II. Bucala, Richard, editor of
compilation.
  [DNLM: 1. Malaria--prevention & control. 2. Malaria--history. WC 765]
  RA644.M2
  362.1969'362--dc23
                                                                    2013030749

British Library Cataloguing-in-Publication Data
A catalogue record for this book is available from the British Library.

In-house Editor: Darilyn Yap

Typeset by Stallion Press
Email: enquiries@stallionpress.com

Printed in Singapore

Contents

Introduction

Frank M. Snowden and Richard Bucala

Malaria is one of the most important "emerging" or "resurgent" infectious diseases. According to the World Health Organization, this mosquito-borne infection is a leading cause of suffering, death, poverty, and underdevelopment in the world today. In 2010, 220 million people contracted malaria, and at least 660,000 died — the great majority of them women and children under five living in sub-Saharan Africa. It is estimated that a child dies of the disease every sixty seconds, making malaria — together with HIV/AIDS and tuberculosis — a leading public health emergency.

The burden of malaria, however, is heavier than statistics for mortality and morbidity indicate. It is a terrible complication of pregnancy, leading to high rates of miscarriage, of maternal death through hemorrhage and severe anemia, and of all the sequelae that follow from severe low birth weight. Since malaria can be transmitted transplacentally from mother to fetus, it can also lead to the birth of infants who are congenitally infected. Furthermore, malaria is a major immuno-suppressive disease, and its victims are therefore highly susceptible to other diseases, especially respiratory infections such as tuberculosis, influenza, and pneumonia. In those areas of the tropical world where malaria is hyperendemic and transmission continues throughout the year, the population at risk can be infected, reinfected or superinfected every year. If they survive, the victims possess a painfully acquired partial immunity, but it comes at a high and enduring cost because repeated bouts of malaria often lead to severe neurological deficit and cognitive impairment. The results are ineradicable poverty, illiteracy, compromised economic growth, a stunted development of civil society, and political instability. In the words of Ronald Ross, the Nobel Prize laureate who discovered the mosquito theory of transmission, malaria enslaves those it does not kill. Malaria is a major contributor to the inequalities between North and South, and of the dependency of the Third World. The direct costs of the disease are estimated at US $12 billion per year.

This situation of contemporary crisis is paradoxical because the early decades following the Second World War marked a period of unrestrained optimism in the international scientific and public health communities. In part, this optimism was a reflection of a generalized medical hubris. By the 1950s, medical science seemed to be on the verge of a final triumph over all communicable diseases. Vaccines promised the elimination from the globe of smallpox, diphtheria, and polio; public health infrastructures such as sewage systems, the sand filtration and chlorination of water, and the pasteurization of milk suggested the conquest of water and foodborne scourges such as cholera, typhoid, salmonellosis, and dysentery; the discovery of the antibiotics penicillin and streptomycin suggested the end of tuberculosis and syphilis; and the discovery of powerful new pesticides led many to predict the swift end of vectorborne diseases, including malaria, dengue fever, sleeping sickness, typhus, and yellow fever. Communicable diseases, it was believed, were on the verge of being eradicated from the globe, one by one. In the words of the Surgeon-General of the United States in 1969, the time had come to close the book on infectious diseases. Alberto Missiroli, the Italian High Commissioner for Health, envisaged the return of humans to an insect-free Eden in which all contagious diseases had been eliminated. Similarly, E. Harold Hinman wrote a book entitled *World Eradication of Infectious Diseases.* This unbridled euphoria produced the theory of the "Disease Transition," which gave analytical rigor to Missiroli's vision. It held that the world stood on the point of escaping the long millennia of plagues and pestilence in order to enter an era when the only diseases to afflict mankind would be chronic and degenerative ailments — above all, heart disease and cancer.

The disease that initiated this postwar optimism was malaria, thanks to the development of an apparent panacea — DDT. The most influential proponent of DDT was Paul Russell, the eminent Rockefeller malariologist, who published in 1955 *Man's Mastery of Malaria,* in which he proclaimed the "DDT era of malariology" and predicted a swift global victory over the ancient scourge. Adopting Russell's optimism as policy, the eighth World Health Assembly meeting in Mexico City in May 1955 launched an unprecedented and ambitious campaign of worldwide eradication based on the power of the new weapon and its standardized four-stage program of "preparation, attack, consolidation, and maintenance."

Unfortunately, the heady vision of 1955 rapidly ran into insoluble difficulties. Mosquitoes rapidly developed resistance to the organochlorine. In addition, the political will needed to provide adequate funds for the project and to overcome the inevitable difficulties it encountered proved inadequate. Paradoxically, the very announcement of an easy and rapid victory undermined the campaign by discouraging researchers, donors, and physicians from entering a field that was so soon to become redundant. The malarial problem revealed itself to be far more intractable than the DDT enthusiasts had imagined. By the end of the 1960s, the idea of global eradication had become a mirage that was as distant as ever, and the entire program collapsed in disillusionment and confusion.

After 1969, the crisis deepened. A variety of factors tipped the balance in favor of the parasites and the mosquitoes that serve as their vectors. These factors include the development of drug resistant *Plasmodia*; wars, migrant labor, and the displacement of people; the synergy between malaria and the co-epidemics of HIV/AIDS and tuberculosis; development projects such as building dams and clearing forests that have degraded the environment and created opportunities for *anophelines*; the adaptation of such major vectors as *Anopheles gambiae* to urban habitats; climate change that has favored the breeding of mosquitoes; and the persistence of poverty and substandard housing that place humans at risk from arthropods. Instead of disappearing, malaria is resurgent.

The Global Challenge of Malaria: Past Lessons and Future Prospects examines malaria from an interdisciplinary and transnational perspective. The idea for the book began with an international conference held at Yale University in November 2008. The unusual feature of this was that it brought together experts on the disease from a variety of disciplines and perspectives — physicians, research scientists, historians of medicine, public health officials, and representatives of several NGOs — who pooled their knowledge and experience to assess the strengths and weaknesses of past efforts at malaria control, and then to draft practical recommendations that could be helpfully borne in mind in present and future antimalarial campaigns, particularly in Africa. The recommendations grew directly out of the presentations and discussions during the three days at Yale, and they were offered in the hope of assisting those involved in the process of ameliorating this scourge of humanity.

Fortunately, even as the conference met, there were hopeful signs of progress in the struggle. Awareness has grown of the appalling magnitude of the burden of sickness and death caused by malaria and its complications and sequelae. There is a wave of financial support for the application of already known control measures and for research to devise new tools. Global mortality by 2011 had fallen by a quarter since the turn of the new century. In this still somber but less despairing context, there is an urgent need to use all available resources in a rational and integrated strategy to reduce the unacceptable suffering caused by a disease that is both treatable and preventable. As these efforts are made, it is vital to remember that significant efforts at malaria eradication have been made in the past, and that unrealistic goals, unsustainable methodologies, and neglect of the lessons of history all too often led to a severe backlash of despair and disillusionment.

As a result of our deliberations at the Symposium, the participants recommended measures to ensure that resources are deployed effectively and that vital lessons of earlier eradication and control efforts are integrated into the antimalarial campaign of the international community. These recommendations were:

(1) The President's Malaria Initiative (PMI) should appoint a board of experienced advisers, including experts with historical knowledge and experts on malaria in Africa. As an internationally recognized organization of specialists, the American Society of Tropical Medicine and Hygiene should also appoint an advisory panel of persons with relevant experience of malaria control. The advice of this panel should be offered to the PMI and the NGOs in the field. We further suggest that NGOs involved in the antimalarial campaign appoint boards of experienced and historically informed advisers to oversee their programs and make recommendations. An understanding of past malaria control efforts is important if earlier mistakes are to be avoided.

(2) All antimalarial efforts should be tailored to the specific needs of individual countries, taking due account of their health infrastructure, epidemiology, ecology, and political realities. Inevitably, success will depend strongly on national stability and economic health. The long-term goal of PMI and other outside institutions should be to shift implementation to indigenous institutions such as National Malaria Control Programs, which will require support and augmentation by PMI and other funding agencies.

(3) Research aimed at the development of new tools in the struggle such as vaccines, vector control technologies, and medications should be adequately funded in an ongoing manner, but without delaying the rational use of already available methodologies.

(4) Planning should empower individuals, local authorities, and national health ministers by educating them about malaria. Top-down and one-size-fits-all approaches must be carefully avoided.

(5) A vital function of the health infrastructure must be the rigorous monitoring of mosquitoes, parasite prevalence, and other malariometric indices. These locally collected data should be the basis for planning and for evaluating results. The PMI and other agencies involved in malaria control should establish and strengthen national laboratories with trained and qualified local staff to generate this information for local use.

(6) There should be no illusion of rapid success against malaria, perhaps the oldest of human diseases, because unrealistic targets and unsustainable goals carry the dangers of fatalism and the abandonment of the effort. Once begun, the campaign must be sustained. Otherwise there is the risk that temporary but unsustainable advances could have unanticipated, negative consequences. These could include promoting mosquito and parasite resistance and compromising acquired immunity. Devastating epidemics could then ensue as has

happened in the past. Strategies setting priorities should be gradually developed into long-term public health efforts that can be maintained at regional levels rather than dramatic but temporary interventions. Sustainability is critical.

(7) The capacity of the World Health Organization to coordinate multilateral efforts and to support national control programs should be strengthened and made effective.

Past efforts at controlling and eliminating malaria have been undermined by poorly designed development projects, armed conflicts, population dislocations, the inability of resource-poor nations to sustain control programs, and levels of poverty that prevent populations from having access to preventive or curative measures. Successful malaria control and elimination demand tremendous patience, vision, and long-term commitment.

The chapters that follow embody much of the thinking that led to these conclusions although the participants in the conference and the contributors to this volume are not identical. Part I consists of historical reflections on significant attempts, both successful and failed, to deal with malaria in different geographical conditions. Margaret Humphreys analyzes the history of malaria in the United States from the introduction of the disease until its final eradication; Darwin Stapleton studies the insecticidal approach to malaria control by the Rockefeller Foundation from 1920 to 1950; James Webb assesses pilot studies for the WHO global eradication campaign after World War II; Frank Snowden discusses the Sardinian Project of 1946–1951 that was a prototype for the global effort; and Socrates Litsios considers the inadequate role of popular education in malaria control efforts.

Part II considers malaria more from the contemporary scientific, medical, and public health perspectives. Brian Greenwood deals with the role of The Gambia in scientific research; Harry Flaster, Emily Mosites, and Brian Blackburn assess the role of insecticide-treated bednets in malaria control; and Tiffany Sun and Richard Bucala consider the challenges of malaria to the medical and scientific communities.

Acknowledgements

The Contributors would like to thank all of those who assisted them in the preparation of these chapters. Our combined intellectual, financial, and personal debts are far too lengthy to be listed here, but we thank all of those who have assisted each of us in his/her individual work. This book would not have appeared without their generosity. In addition, we wish as a group, to acknowledge our appreciation for the financial assistance provided by the provost's office at Yale University, which made possible the original conference from which this book emerged.

Contributors

Brian G. Blackburn
MD, Clinical Associate Professor of Medicine, Division of Infectious Diseases and Geographic Medicine, Stanford University School of Medicine

Richard Bucala
MD, PhD, Professor of Medicine, Pathology, Epidemiology & Public Health, Yale University

Harry V. Flaster
MD, Stanford University School of Medicine

Brian Greenwood
MD, PhD, Professor of Clinical Tropical Medicine, Faculty of Infectious and Tropical Diseases, London School of Hygiene & Tropical Medicine

Margaret Humphreys
MD, PhD, Josiah Charles Trent Professor in the History of Medicine, Duke University School of Medicine

Socrates Litsios
PhD, Retired Senior Scientist, Division of Control of Tropical Diseases, World Health Organization

Emily Mosites
MPH, Vectorbourne Disease Section, Tennessee Department of Health

Frank M. Snowden
PhD, Andrew Downey Orrick Professor of History, Yale University

Darwin H. Stapleton
PhD, Professor of History, University of Massachusetts

Tiffany Sun
PhD, Yale School of Medicine, Yale University

James L. Webb, Jr.
PhD, Professor of History, Colby College

Part I

Lessons of History

1   Malaria in America

Margaret Humphreys

Introduction

Malaria was once a major cause of illness and death in the United States, although it is now almost entirely limited to imported cases arriving from other countries where the disease persists.[1] By 1950, home-grown malaria had disappeared in the United States, as well as in other temperate countries such as England, Holland, Spain, and Italy. Their stories of eradication make tempting models for those seeking to control a disease that still sickens and kills millions of people in the world today, most of them living in tropical and sub-tropical environments. As major new initiatives in the twenty-first century once again take on the microscopic predator carried in the mosquito's spittle, it is worth asking whether history can offer lessons that can guide the effort.

Ten years ago I concluded that historical research on malaria in the United States bore no "relevance for the beleaguered international malarial community," as the story contained "no startling revelations about how to fight malaria," and instead described methods and processes already well known to malaria campaigners.[2] In retrospect, I have come to conclude that this assessment was too modest. George Santayana, in a now famous comment concerning history, said "Those who cannot remember the past, are condemned to repeat it."[3] While the history of malaria in the United States offers no simple solutions for today's malaria challenges, it does contain lessons that those designing modern malaria wars would do well to keep in mind. Although no one now thinks, as optimistic malariologists did in the 1950s, that the victory over malaria in the United States and Europe which

---

[1] This paper's title uses "America" in its common colloquial sense in the U.S., to refer to the colonies and states that ultimately formed the modern U.S.

[2] Margaret Humphreys, *Malaria: Poverty, Race and Public Health in the United States*, The Johns Hopkins University Press, 2001, 6: Baltimore, London.

[3] George Santayana, *The Life of Reason, or Phases of Human Progress*, Charles Scribner's Sons, 1905, 5 vols., 284: New York.

had been won with DDT and chloroquine could be easily duplicated elsewhere, it is important to sort out the geographical, economic, social and political differences that contributed to malaria's demise in the developed western countries in order to recognize how the possible interventions available then and now interact with these various factors.

This chapter will first briefly outline malaria's history in the United States, focusing particularly on several points along the way when malaria escalated or declined, with the goal of identifying the key causes of such expansion and contraction. It will then conclude with the policy implications that are suggested by this story.

The Parasites and Their Vectors

Although the label malaria is commonly used as if it were a single disease, there are actually four malaria parasites in humans that cause four different diseases. Only three were common in the United States, and for simplicity's sake can be divided into severe (*falciparum*) malaria and milder (*vivax* and *malariae*) malaria. *Falciparum* can be deadly, especially when newly introduced to a population. Philip Curtin found that white British troops garrisoned on the west coast of Africa had a mortality rate in one year of over 50%; while other diseases such as yellow fever contributed to this slaughter, *falciparum* was the major culprit.[4] *Vivax* is milder, and probably kills less than 5% of its victims, even without the benefit of curative drugs. *Malariae* seems to have had a minor presence in the United States, and for general purposes can be considered as similar to *vivax*.[5] The parasites destroy red blood cells, leading to anemia and weakness. The spleen grows increasingly palpable as it struggles to clean up the destroyed red blood cells of the infected host. *Falciparum* malaria is more deadly because its parasites multiply in such massive numbers that they clog the capillaries of kidney, brain and liver, leading to failure of those essential organs. The *vivax* and *falciparum* organisms tend to cycle in and out of the red cells every 48 hours, giving the disease its

---

[4]Philip D. Curtin, *Death by Migration: Europe's Encounter with the tropical World in the Nineteenth Century*, Cambridge University Press, 1989: Cambridge.

[5]Malarial diseases have gone under many names. *Vivax* and *falciparum* cycle through red cells every 48 hours, so earned the names benign tertian malaria and malignant tertian malaria, respectively. Tertian referred to the appearance of symptoms every third day. These diseases might also be labeled by their predominating seasonal appearance, with *vivax* more common in the spring and *falciparum* in the fall, at least in the sub-tropical climates of the United States; *malariae* had a quartan, or every fourth day cycle. Microscopes were not common in the American south during the years malaria prevailed there, and usually only researchers doing special studies had the equipment and the skills to precisely diagnose malaria based on blood smears.

common name in the nineteenth century, intermittent fever. And when the fever spikes, it causes severe chills, shaking and fever, a miserable agitation that may be related to the other common name for malaria, ague.[6]

Both diseases are particularly harsh to children and pregnant women. The malaria parasites compromise the placental blood supply, leading to miscarriage and stillbirth, while the mother's normal decrease in immune surveillance during pregnancy makes her particularly vulnerable to the disease. On the other hand, those people that grow up in an environment of endemic malaria acquire tolerance to the organisms over time. Populations that have lived for millennia with the malaria parasites (and since the higher primates all have their own malarias, it is likely that the relationship goes back to the dawn of humans in Africa) have developed various hereditary traits that all attempt to make the red blood cell less susceptible to the invading parasite. Hence the sickle cell trait, G6PD deficiency, hemoglobin C trait, and the various thallasemias all appear to protect children against *falciparum* malaria. Many Africans also lack the Duffy antigen on the wall of their red cells, a benign mutation that protects them entirely from illness by the *vivax* organism. While the humans that left Africa to migrate to other parts of Europe and Asia probably included malaria carriers, it is likely that the disease died out in the small scattered bands of migrants, only to be reintroduced by trade after population growth.[7]

The predominant "malaria mosquito" in the United States was *Anopheles quadrimaculatus* (*A. quad.*), a mosquito distributed broadly from the east coast to the middle of the country, and from Florida into lower Canada. The mosquito identified as *A. quad.* by malariologists in the mid-twentieth century has now been recognized to be a species complex, a phrase used to designate a cluster of mosquito types that may be designated sub-species by some and separate species by others. For details on these discussions, see the modern literature on genomics and

---

[6]This information about malaria is widely available in textbooks and online. See, for example, Rick M. Fairhurst and Thomas E. Wellems, *Plasmodium* Species (Malaria), in Gerald Mandell, John Bennett, and Raphael Dolin, eds., *Mandell, Douglas and Bennett's Principles and Practice of Infectious Disease*, 7th ed., Elsevier/Churchill Livingstone, 2009, **2**, 275: New York, available online at http://www.mdconsult.com/book. *Plasmodium knowlesi* is another malaria parasite that can infect humans. It was thought to be primarily an infection of apes, but has recently been found widespread in humans in Southeast Asia. It can be easily confused with *Plasmodium malariae*. Whether it ever occurred indigenously in the United States is unknown but unlikely, given its limited geographic distribution today. See J. Cox-Singh *et al.*, *Plasmodium knowlesi* malaria in humans is widely distributed and potentially life threatening, *Clinical Infectious Diseases,* 2008, **46**, 165–71 for a description of *Plasmodium knowlesi* infection in Malaysia.

[7]D. J. Weatherall, Common genetic disorders of the red cell and the 'Malaria Hypothesis', *Annals of Tropical Medicine and Parasitology,* 1987, **81**, 539–48.

distribution.[8] For our purposes, the simple name will do, and the mosquito's characteristics that are relevant to malaria transmission can be briefly described. First, *A. quad.* is a "promiscuous" feeder — malariologists dissected *A. quads.* from various states in the American south and found that mosquitoes trapped in environments where farm animals and people were equally available showed no preference in their choice of blood meal.[9] Erwin Ackerknecht has argued that malaria retreated from the upper Mississippi Valley in part because as the number of farm animals increased, the mosquitoes chose them for feeding over humans.[10] This does not seem to have been the case in the south, and may explain in part the persistence of malaria in that region. *Anopheles freeborni* was the predominant vector of malaria on the west coast, especially in California.[11]

The major malaria vectors in the United States breed in still water, preferring swamps, ponds, and side pools of moving streams for laying their eggs. Once hatched, the mosquitoes rarely fly more than a mile from their breeding site, so malaria cases clustered around such wetlands. Malaria larvae float on the surface of the water, where they are susceptible to consumption by small fish, poisoning by larvicides, or smothering by a layer of oil.

Immigrants to the New World and the Arrival of Malaria

The migrants who settled in the area which would become the United States came from four major areas. First, the Native Americans arrived in prehistoric times, and

---

[8]Rebecca S. Levine, A. Townsend Peterson, and Mark Q. Benedict, Distribution of members of *Anopheles quadrimaculatus* Say s.l. (Diptera: Culicidae) and implications for their roles in malaria transmission in the United States, *Journal of Medical Entomology*, 2004, **41**, 607–13; Robert F. Darsie Jr. and Ronald A. Ward, *Identification and Geographical Distribution of the Mosquitoes of North America, North of Mexico*, University Press of Florida, 2005: Gainesville. While other *Anopheles* species may have been locally important, *A. quad.* was the predominant malaria mosquito in the American South. James Stevens Simmons reviewed the research on malaria vectors in the United States in, The Transmission of Malaria by *Anopheles* Mosquitoes in North America, in Forest Ray Moultin, ed., *A Symposium on Human Malaria with Special Reference to North America and the Caribbean Region*, American Association for the Advancement of Science, 1941, 113–30: Washington.
[9]F.W. O'Connor, Biologic investigations, *Southern Medical Journal*, 1924, **17**, 599–602; S.T. Darling, Discussion on the relative importance in transmitting malaria of *Anopheles Quadrimaculatus*, *Punctipennis*, and *Crucians* and advisability of differentiating between these species in applying control measures, *Southern Medical Journal*, 1925, **18**, 452–8; and S.T. Darling, Entomological research in malaria, *Southern Medical Journal*, 1925, **18**, 446–9.
[10]Erwin H. Ackerknecht, *Malaria in the Upper Mississippi Valley, 1760–1900*, Arno Press, 1977, c1945: New York.
[11]Simmons, Transmission of Malaria, and Mark F. Boyd, *An Introduction to Malariology*, Harvard University Press, 1930: Cambridge.

appear to have been malaria-free until European settlement. The second group came from the various countries of Europe and the Mediterranean, and many of them would have brought *vivax* parasites along, as this organism is particularly adept at traveling. It can lie dormant in the liver for months, and later cause relapses which start a new cycle of infection wherever the unlucky victim may have roamed in the interim. The third population came from the west coast of Africa, when slave traders imported not only unfortunate humans but the parasites of malaria and, later, yellow fever. Africans were vehicles mainly for *falciparum*, since they were largely immune to *vivax*. Where Africans were forcibly settled and the climate was sufficiently sub-tropical, *falciparum* malaria blossomed in the settlements of the New World colonies. It is possible that immigrants from Asia contributed to the malaria prevalence on the west coasts of North, Central and South America during the last millennia.[12]

Falciparum malaria exploded most evidently in colonial South Carolina, where slave workers harvested rice from flooded fields that were ideal for breeding the *anopheles* species that carry the parasite from one person to another. The impact on mortality, particularly among whites, was so evident that we can pinpoint it fairly precisely, to the early 1680s.[13] From being a fairly healthy colony, South Carolina became deadly for white people. Not coincidentally, the slave trade from the Caribbean and Africa expanded dramatically in just the same time period.[14] One historian who studied South Carolina parish records for the eighteenth century found that 86% of white babies born in some parishes died before the age of 20, an astounding outcome likely due in large measure to *falciparum* malaria. It was no accident that well into the nineteenth century South Carolina had more black people than white, and that planter rhetoric proclaimed that only black people were physically suited to plantation work.[15] White southerners learned to take their families to the Appalachian highlands or northern retreats during the late summer months when the heat was so unpleasant and deadly malaria prevailed.

Fortunately for white settlers in the lands that were to become the United States, *falciparum* did not tolerate the temperatures much further north than Tennessee and North Carolina. *Vivax*, on the other hand, was quite adapted to temperate

---

[12] Humphreys, *Malaria, op. cit.*, 20–6.

[13] Peter Wood, *Black Majority: Negroes in Colonial South Carolina from 1670 through the Stono Rebellion*, Alfred A. Knopf, 1974, 63–91: New York.

[14] Philip Curtin, Epidemiology and the slave trade, *Political Science Quarterly*, 1968, **83**, 191–216.

[15] Peter Coclanis, *The Shadow of a Dream: Economic Life and Death in the South Carolina Low Country, 1670–1920*, Oxford University Press, 1989: New York; H. Roy Merrens and George D. Terry, Dying in paradise: malaria, mortality, and the perceptual environment in colonial South Carolina, *The Journal of Southern History*, 1984, **50**, 533–50.

climes, and extended as far north as Ontario and New Hampshire, and as far west as Iowa, Minnesota and Nebraska. Malaria made life miserable on the American frontier, as so much travel was by river and the earliest settlements were near those transportation waterways. Frontier housing was porous, and mill ponds (created to grind the ubiquitous corn that fed the pioneers and their animals) formed ideal nurseries for *anopheles* larvae. Malaria wreaked havoc in the 18th century Chesapeake, and in the Connecticut River Valley; by the mid-nineteenth century it had traveled into the Midwest, following settlers on the Ohio, the Mississippi and the Missouri Rivers. By the time of the Civil War, both *vivax* and *falciparum* malaria were well entrenched in the United States, although by then it had become rare in New England.

Conditions during the war vastly amplified malaria's spread among Americans. Whereas pest mosquitoes and notions of ill health had kept some areas sparsely populated, soldiers had to camp and fight in places they would otherwise have avoided. The James River peninsula, the shores of the Potomac River, the swamps around Vicksburg, and the occupation of the southern low country all brought men, malaria parasites, and mosquitoes together in great numbers. And those men were living outdoors, with only the slight protection of a tent to ward off mosquitoes. At times troops were issued mosquito netting in particularly buggy locations, but for most Civil War soldiers, these were an absent luxury. Of the several million men who served as soldiers in the war, at least a third on both sides sickened with malaria and 1 to 3% of those ill died of the disease. It was a major cause of disability during the conflict, even when it was not fatal.[16]

Fighting Back

By the mid-nineteenth century, humans began to fight back against malaria with increasing success. In 1821 Parisian researchers Joseph Pelletier and Joseph Caventou isolated quinine from the bark of the cinchona tree, and by the 1840s quinine pills were widely available on the malarious American frontier.[17] As that frontier became more prosperous, settlers built houses more impervious to the

---

[16]*The Medical and Surgical History of the War of the Rebellion, (1861–1865)*, Prepared, in Accordance with Acts of Congress, under the Direction of Surgeon General Joseph K. Barnes, United States Army, Government Printing Office, 1870, 636–7: Washington. And see, Andrew Bell, *Mosquito Soldiers: Malaria, Yellow Fever and the Course of the American Civil War*, Louisiana State University Press, 2010: Baton Rouge.

[17]Dale C. Smith, Quinine and fever: the development of the effective dosage, *Journal of the History of Medicine and Allied Sciences*, 1976, **31**, 343–67; Thomas Findley, Sappington's anti-fever pills and the Westward migration, *Transactions of the American Clinical and Climatological Association*, 1968, **79**, 34–44.

cold, and moved to higher ground where mosquito pests were less abusive. Drainage to ready land for agriculture decreased breeding sites. With the spread of railroads from the 1830s and 1840s, settlers lost their dependence on waterways for transport. All of these actions began to cut malaria rates, especially in the more temperate northern tier of states. The Civil War temporarily reversed this trend, as veterans brought the parasite home and areas such as western New England that had not seen malaria in decades were again affected.[18] But by 1900 malaria had become largely a disease of the south, with a few outposts on the west coast and in the southernmost parts of the midwest.[19]

Whereas prior theorists had declared that malaria emerged from the stinky air of swampy lands, scientists working in the last two decades of the nineteenth century identified the *plasmodium* and demonstrated its carriage by the *anopheles* mosquito. These discoveries quickly generated new tools for fighting the disease. Mosquito larvae could be killed by oiling breeding grounds or sprinkling the water with toxic chemicals. Where possible, drainage removed the breeding sites altogether. Public health officials also recognized that giving quinine to patients or even prophylactically to a whole community would reduce the parasite burden of individuals and decrease transmission. William Crawford Gorgas was able to control both malaria and yellow fever in the Panama Canal Zone, given the power and infusion of enough money to effectively control mosquitoes and treat patients.[20]

These measures were implemented to protect American military camps during World War I, and tested in demonstration projects run by the Rockefeller Foundation in the Mississippi Delta in the post-war years. The Rockefeller Foundation recognized that malaria was most problematic in tropical and subtropical parts of the world that were marked by poverty. It sought to determine which method of malaria control was both the cheapest and most effective. Their demonstration projects targeted this objective, judging the results by cost per case of malaria reduced. They supplied free quinine at one site, organized larvicidal measures at a second, and sponsored a screening campaign at the third.

In the screening campaign, the Rockefeller men and local public health officials enlisted high school shop classes to make simple screens for doors and windows.

---

[18] Francis A. Walker, *Statistical Atlas of the United States Based on the Results of the Ninth Census 1870: with Contributions from Many Eminent Men of Science and Several Departments of the Government*, Julius Bien, 1874, facs. rpt. Ross Pub, 2003: New York, plate XLII (unpaginated).

[19] Linda Nash discusses malaria in California's Central Valley in *Inescapable Ecologies: A History of Environment, Disease and Knowledge*, University of California Press, 2006: Berkeley.

[20] On the general history of this era and the development of new measures of malaria control based on parasite and mosquito vector, see Gordon Harrison, *Mosquitoes, Malaria and Man: A History of the Hostilities since 1880*, E.P. Dutton, 1978: New York, and Randall M. Packard, *The Making of a Tropical Disease: A Short History of Malaria*, The Johns Hopkins University Press, 2007: Baltimore.

They sent educators around to households to demonstrate the installation and maintenance of the screens, and advise on covering wall cracks with heavy brown paper, such as that used for grocery bags. Screens at the time were not rust free, and had to be painted frequently, as well as repaired if holes developed. The program worked well in the first year. In fact every intervention they made worked well in the first year, reducing malaria cases by 90% or more. But then the programs began to fall apart. Physicians objected to the distribution of free medication as impinging on their right to practice. And the drug method failed to prevent recurrence in the long term. The second year when surveyors came back to the screened households, they found many of the screens in disrepair. Often the household occupants had changed, as the sharecropping population was so migratory, leaving one farm at the end of a contract for another, hoping for a better deal. The new occupants knew nothing about the program, and had failed to continue maintenance. Others who had heard the first year's lessons found the screens reduced airflow into the stifling cabins, and so stopped using them.

It was the larvicidal program that seemed to work best. It did not depend on the cooperation of the larger population, but instead on the determination of the local authorities who oiled standing water, sprinkled arsenical larvicides on streams and ponds, or diverted waterways into underground culverts. Such work was popular in urban areas, where local officials reaped political acclaim by both reducing malaria and the presence of mosquito pests. Drained land had greater value in the urban setting as well. Although the disease spiked briefly in the counties affected during the 1927 Mississippi River flood, by the early 1930s, malaria was at a low ebb in the United States, and had largely been controlled in urban settings where the benefit of mosquito pest control coupled with public health efforts justify public expenditures on drainage and larvicidal treatments. The affluent had also learned the value of screening their houses, a feature that became increasingly common and expected among the middle class.[21]

The Great Depression temporarily reversed this trend of malaria decline. Many of those who had worked in town returned to the rural countryside, where malaria still thrived. This last surge of the disease in the United States peaked between 1933 and 1935; it had largely disappeared by the early 1940s.[22] The causes of its demise are hard to measure, for a variety of reasons. First, most of the statistics available concern malaria death rates, whereas the number of cases would be a

[21] Humphreys, *Malaria, op. cit.*, 72–87. See also Hoyt Bleakley, Malaria eradication in the Americas: a retrospective analysis of childhood exposure, *American Economic Journal: Applied,* April 2010, **2**(2), 1–45 available from: http://home.uchicago.edu/~bleakley/.
[22] Ernest Carroll Faust, Clinical and public health aspects of malaria in the United States from a historical perspective, *American Journal of Tropical Medicine*, 1945, **25**, 185–201.

much better metric for malaria prevalence (but was rarely collected). Deaths among the rural southern poor were not usually observed by a physician, so the cause of death listed officially was only a guess generated by the family report and the public official creating the death certificate. When the federal public health officials began paying for documented cases (demonstrated by a positive microscopic blood smear examination) in the late 1940s, they found that counties thought to be persistently malarious actually had no cases at all. Individual physician statements about the prevalence of malaria may be more accurate than the official statistics.[23]

It does seem clear that malaria was hard to find by 1940. At Charity Hospital in Louisiana, a malaria case was an exciting event by 1942; instructors made sure that medical students had a chance to see the rare cases. The United States Public Health Service had set up a field station to study malaria in Newton, Georgia in the 1920s, but by 1944 they converted their mission to studying mosquitoes as malaria had disappeared.[24] So what happened in the last half of the 1930s to squash the malaria parasite in the United States? It would be easy to give credit to a region-wide Works Progress Administration program that built drainage systems, including in malarious areas. But this work was poorly planned, not specifically targeted at malarious breeding sites, and offered no systematic plan for maintenance, which meant the drainage ditches quickly clogged and became ineffective (or even increased the water surface for larvae).[25] This was also an era when the Tennessee Valley Authority, Duke Power Company, and other power companies were damming rivers for hydroelectric power. They recognized the capacity of their reservoirs to increase mosquito breeding and hence malaria, and took active steps to control the disease. Their work was limited to the immediate environs of their reservoirs, however, and had little impact on malaria elsewhere, such as in the Mississippi delta region.

The most likely cause for the decline of malaria in these years was an inadvertent by-product of New Deal legislation that sought to improve southern agriculture. Government programs paid farmers to take their land out of cultivation, in order to prop up the prices of the crops that were produced. Federal loan programs supplied capital for farmers to buy machinery such as tractors and other mechanical devices. These measures in turn meant that the old system of sharecropping, in which poor blacks and whites lived in shacks on the land and cultivated it with a

---

[23] Margaret Humphreys, Kicking a dying dog: DDT and the demise of malaria in the American South, 1942–1952, *Isis, 1996,* **87**, 1–17.

[24] Humphreys, Kicking a dying dog, *op. cit.*

[25] Margaret Humphreys, Water won't run uphill: the new deal and malaria control in the American South, 1933–1940. *Parassitologia,* 1998, **40**, 183–92.

hand plow and mule, became less cost effective. A massive depopulation of the southern rural landscape followed, and even where planters hired day labor, that labor lived in town (where malaria had already been controlled). As a result, large populations were removed from the one-mile flight zone around many malaria breeding sites, breaking the chain of malaria transmission.[26]

World War II and New Tools for the Malaria Wars

As the United States entered the world war late in 1941, malaria was not a major problem in the American south. Yet, military and civilian public health leaders feared an upsurge in the disease. They saw malaria as a disease of mysterious cycles, of peaks and troughs of unexplained pattern. With so many military camps in the south, troops from all over the country were at risk as the country mobilized for the war. The United States Public Health Service created a special agency to protect military sites from malaria, and dubbed it Malaria Control in War Areas (MCWA). The military authorities created malaria control programs within military camps, and MCWA's job was to create a malaria free zone around camps and other war-related sites. They used familiar tools — larvicide via oil and arsenic compounds, spraying insecticides containing pyrethrum, screens, insect repellants, and oral medication. Since Japan had occupied Java, where almost all of the world's quinine-source trees now grew, the United States authorities substituted with the drug atabrine. Atabrine was not particularly popular given its side-effect profile, but it kept men on their feet in malaria zones overseas and on American soil.

Two new weapons for the malaria wars emerged from American military research during World War II. The first was the synthesis of chloroquine, a new malaria drug that was far better tolerated than earlier malaria compounds.[27] The second was DDT (dichlorodiphenyltrichloroethane). DDT was a near magical insecticide. Pyrethrum had been used for years, but it was a "knock-down" insecticide, one that killed a mosquito if sprayed directly on it. It had no residual effect. DDT, on the other hand, could be sprayed on a wall and continue killing mosquitoes that landed there for up to three months. It was equally effective as a larvicide, and could be spread on lakes from airplanes or from boats with motorized sprayers. DDT had a major impact on the military control of malaria (and other insect-borne diseases) overseas, and in August 1945 it became available for purchase within the United States.[28]

---

[26]Humphreys, *Malaria, op. cit.*, 108–12.

[27]Leo B. Slater, *War and Disease: Biomedical Research on Malaria in the Twentieth Century*, Rutgers University Press, 2009: New Brunswick.

[28]Edmund Russell, *War and Nature: Fighting Humans and Insects with Chemicals from World War I to Silent Spring*, Cambridge University Press, 2001: New York.

There was one attempt at a controlled study of DDT as an anti-malarial agent in the United States, which focused on an area surrounding two new reservoirs in South Carolina, components of the Santee-Cooper hydroelectric plant project. As one MCWA leader noted in 1945, "The Santee-Cooper offers what may be the last opportunity in this country to see active malaria."[29] He strongly supported a quick research program there to test the effectiveness of DDT. A combined federal and state research team sprayed one area with DDT and left another as a control, but found that malaria declined rapidly among both populations, leading to an inconclusive result.[30]

At the end of the war MCWA had more than four thousand employees, but no longer had a mandate to protect the war effort. Its leaders argued successfully to Congress that agency funding be continued, and they launched a malaria eradication campaign in the United States, using DDT as their principal weapon. Changing their name to the Communicable Disease Center (CDC), MCWA officials oversaw the DDT spraying of millions of homes in the American south from 1945 to 1950.[31] There was very little malaria to measure, so they instead counted the reduction in *Anopheles* mosquitoes, which was significant. In 1951 they declared victory; after a three century run, malaria was no longer indigenous in the United States.[32] It is likely that the CDC campaign eradicated a few remaining pockets of the disease, and deserves some credit for that result. It is also likely that malaria had largely subsided by the time the campaign began, so that their victory was not a difficult one.[33]

There are still about 1,500 cases of malaria cases in the United States each year. Over the past half century, malaria has spread from imported cases to local inhabitants at least 63 times, although the outbreaks have been quite limited.[34] Some have questioned whether with global warming and increased possibilities for the international spread of disease, the United States might be at risk for the re-emer-

[29] L. L. Williams to Alex G. Gilliam, 13 March 1945, Louis L. Williams Papers, 1927–1970, MS C 169, box 5, Santee-Cooper Folder (no. 2), History of Medicine Division, National Library of Medicine, Bethesda, MD.

[30] Leo Slater and Margaret Humphreys, Parasites and progress: ethical decision-making and the Santee-Cooper malaria study, 1944–1949, *Perspectives in Biology and Medicine*, 2008, **51**, 103–20.

[31] On the history of the CDC, see Elizabeth W. Etheridge, *Sentinel for Health: A History of the Centers for Disease Control*, University of California Press, 1992: Berkeley.

[32] Justin M. Andrews, Nationwide malaria eradication projects in the Americas: the eradication program in the U.S.A., *Journal of the National Malaria of Society*, 1951, **10**, 99–121.

[33] Humphreys, Kicking a dying dog, *op. cit.*

[34] Data from CDC website at http://www.cdc.gov/malaria/about/facts.html. More information about individual outbreaks can be found in the *Morbidity and Mortality Weekly Report*, also available online at the CDC website.

gence of malaria.[35] Much has changed in the formerly malarious zones of the country that makes this outcome unlikely. First, most homes in the south are air conditioned, and few people are exposed to the volume of mosquito bites that characterized the malaria years. An interesting study on the border of Mexico illustrated this point.

Paul Reiter and his colleagues wondered why dengue fever, a viral disease spread by mosquitoes of the *Aedes* genus, had erupted in Nuevo Laredo, when Laredo, Texas was almost entirely spared. The two cities were only a bridge span apart, and the research team actually found a higher density of the vector in Laredo than on the Mexican side of the border. The key difference between the two communities was air conditioning. Mexicans spent the leisure hours of the early evening, when mosquitoes are most active, outside on patios or in open air bars, whereas most American housing and public places were air conditioned, limiting mosquito exposure.[36] There was no difference in climate between the two communities. The few documented instances where malaria spread locally within the United States in recent years occurred mostly in the lowest grade of housing, such as trailer parks whose residents likewise spent the early evening hours sitting outside their residences. American cities actively control pest mosquitoes, and one assumes that if an outbreak of severe mosquito borne disease did erupt, these measures would correspondingly increase. This has certainly happened in the response to West Nile Virus, an organism spread by mosquitoes, which caused significant disease in certain localities of the United States. It is hard to imagine malaria making a comeback in the modern United States, unless major changes in societal affluence and government infrastructure occur first.[37]

Lessons Learned

It is worth recognizing the factors that first amplified malaria in the United States. First, frontier populations are a prime target for the disease, especially when the mode of transport is by water. Areas of new settlement are characterized by initial poverty, porous housing, subsistence agriculture, and high cost of manufactured goods such as medicines. As humans enter a previously unsettled area, they may alter the landscape in ways that increase mosquito breeding, such as by building

---

[35] Margaret Humphreys, Climate change and mosquito-borne disease: a historical perspective, *MD Advisor*, 2009, **2**, 16–21.

[36] P. Reiter *et al.*, Texas lifestyle limits transmission of dengue virus, *Emerging Infectious Diseases*, 2003, **9**, 1–9.

[37] Information on West Nile Virus is available at http//:www.cdc.gov. According to one report on that site, The state of California voted an extra 12 million dollars for mosquito control in 2005 when West Nile became a major public health threat there.

dams for power. Even when modern tools are available to fight malaria, those living on the frontier fringes may be most susceptible if the malaria parasite is present.

Second, war is a grand amplifier of malaria epidemics. Humans will usually move away from mosquito hordes if they have a choice, since the insects create such misery. Wartime conditions may force the occupation of landscapes that would otherwise be lightly populated, and if the malaria parasite is introduced, it will find dense human populations ripe for mass transmission of the disease. Even with the tools of quinine and mosquito netting available, the American Civil War not only saw the rapid spread of malaria among troops on both sides, but the re-introduction of the disease to areas long free of it. War sets populations in motion, and often creates refugee camps for those fleeing the destruction generated by combat. Populations that may have once lived in villages where malaria was fairly well controlled may be forced into new locales where all of those systems fall apart and they are newly subjected to the disease.

Third, poverty is tied to malaria in multiple ways. Those weakened by malaria are unable to work at full capacity, and their infected children will suffer stunted growth and educational disabilities, perpetuating the impoverishment engendered by malaria. The poor are likely to live in substandard housing, that lacks screens or (in the modern era) the air conditioning that makes life indoors tolerable in tropical climates. This housing may, in turn, increase exposure to mosquitoes (as was the case in the Nuevo Laredo study). It may also make it difficult to institute programs designed to decrease contact between humans and mosquitoes. If shacks are so porous that the inhabitants worry about snakes entering the habitation, screens are likely to have little impact on mosquito entry. For the DDT spraying program of the 1940s to be effective, the population had to live in houses with walls. Populations that live in dwellings that lack even these simple amenities — such as people living in refugee camps, tents, or primitive shacks — may be unreachable by interventions that target mosquitoes via screening or residual spraying.

Poverty also affects access to medication. The malaria peak in the 1930s United States would have been much duller if the population had been able to afford quinine. Doctors bemoaned the fact that the sick did not visit them nor receive effective doses of quinine, and instead spent what money they had on low dose "chill tonics" that contained inadequate amounts of quinine, if any at all. Poor southerners in the Great Depression had very little cash on hand, and effective medicine was out of reach for many. If every American with malaria in the 1930s had access to a doctor and proper medication, the parasite could not have thrived. The onset of the great poverty of that decade demonstrated the impact of economic recession on health, and especially on diseases that had been fairly well controlled when economic conditions had been only slightly better.

The malaria story in the United States offers other lessons as well, lessons about human behavior and the effectiveness of public health education campaigns. The Rockefeller demonstration projects in the Mississippi Delta in the late 1910s showed that just about any viable program (drugs, screens, drainage) would be effective in its first year. But as soon as the fervor of the initial encounter had begun to wane, malaria crept back. This was particularly the case for screening, which relied on the individual to maintain vigilance against damage and persist in proper usage. Modern interventions (such as bed net programs) that require steady maintenance and strict, persistent use in the face of inconvenience or discomfort may be equally likely to succeed, at first, and then fail as the intervention's initial impact fades over time. Failure of malaria programs is particularly problematic, since when the disease returns it finds a population whose acquired immunity has waned. Any malaria control program needs to measure the effect of an intervention over more than one or two years, and be prepared for long term surveillance and continued dedication on the part of local actors.

The decline of cases during the 1930s also demonstrates the importance of location for the prevalence of malaria. Where mosquitoes have a limited flight distance from their breeding grounds, the proximity of people to those breeding sites becomes critical. One study of malaria in an eastern North Carolina village in 1940 showed that proximity to the town's major pond was a more important variable in predicting the occurrence of malaria than the quality of the housing (a marker of affluence).[38] If my research is correct, and the major decline of malaria in the United States occurred because of rural depopulation, then observers considering the American story should be careful in attributing the eradication of malaria to direct measures taken against it. In many tropical countries, it may be impossible to remove people from proximity to *Anopheles* breeding sites. But it would be incorrect to state that "DDT eradicated malaria in the United States, and it ought to be used elsewhere to similar success," an assumption that guided the tropical malaria eradication programs of the 1950s and 1960s, and has some adherents today.

Malaria seems to particularly invite facile but false assumptions about its eradication. Nathan Myhrvold, described as "Bill Gates's ideas guy" told an interviewer for Foreign Policy:

> Malaria is the only disease to ever be locally eradicated without any medicine. It turns out that if you drain the swamps, spray with DDT or other pesticides, put window screens on [the windows], and have a tremendous amount of discipline, you can defeat malaria. That's how it was defeated in the United States in the 1930s. In 1935, the peak year, there were 135,000 cases. This was a furious disease in the southern

---

[38] Humphreys, *Malaria*, *op. cit.*, 110.

United States. We got that fixed. The trouble is, we got that fixed because we had a combination of a high standard of living and a lot of resources and some discipline. The countries that have it worst [with malaria today] have very low standards of living and very little societal discipline. They can't put their effort into malaria right now.[39]

Myhrvold has invented a laser mosquito zapper which he thinks will stop malaria, although he concedes it is more likely to be a commercial success as a backyard insecticide in countries of affluence. His attribution of malaria's disappearance in the United States to discipline, resources, and a high standard of living contains some truth, but he misses the major explanation of its demise. Drawing conclusions based on bad history is poor public policy.

The disappearance of malaria in the United States and Europe during the 1940s led to great global optimism about the possibility of eradicating malaria worldwide. Yet in retrospect there is little evidence that DDT was key in the disappearance of American malaria, and the successful eradication of malaria in temperate climates may have little relevance to tropical areas. Public health campaigners should use care in comparing the events in one locale, with its own peculiar circumstances of climate, populations, housing, and infrastructure, with other areas where key factors may be different. Malaria is easy to control — with enough money and determination — and yet remains one of the major health hazards today, especially for children and pregnant women. The history of campaigns against this slippery antagonist over the past century provides important object lessons for those seeking once again to conquer this disease.[40]

---

[39] Elizabeth Dickinson, The Ultimate Bug Zapper, [an interview with Nathan Myhrvold], *Foreign Policy*, 23 April 2010, available at http://www.foreignpolicy.com/articles/2010/04/23/interview_nathan_myhrvold (accessed on 2 May 2010).

[40] Packard, *The Making of a Tropical Disease, op. cit.*; Socrates Litsios, *The Tomorrow of Malaria*, Pacific Press, 1997: Wellington, NZ.

2 Technological Solutions: The Rockefeller Insecticidal Approach to Malaria Control, 1920–1950

Darwin H. Stapleton

In 2008, the magazine of the Natural Resources Defense Council published an article that focused on the upsurge of malaria in Africa and dealt substantially with the question of insecticide use. A central passage in the article read:

> In September 2006 the World Health Organization issued a press release headlined, "WHO Gives Indoor Use of DDT a Clean Bill of Health for Controlling Malaria." It was a startling announcement, apparently contradicting the position [WHO] had held on DDT since the 1970s.... Five years earlier the Stockholm Convention had sanctioned the use of DDT in prescribed circumstances. DDT tends to be most desperately needed, and most reliable, in epidemic conditions, where the break in the transmission cycle that it provides can be dramatically effective. In such instances, the immediate need to save lives trumps concerns about subsequent health or environmental complications (including the potential for mosquitoes to develop resistance to the toxin). It was recognition of this stark calculus that forged the 2001 compromise on DDT, which was agreed to by groups with histories of firm opposition to the insecticide, such as the World Wildlife Fund, the Natural Resources Defense Council (NRDC), and the Pesticide Action Network (PAN).[1]

This matter-of-fact statement from an avowed opponent of DDT, and virtually all broad-spectrum insecticides, suggests why it is worthwhile to look back into the history of insecticidal approaches to malaria control. It indicates that the most reviled insecticide, DDT, remains effective, indeed "desperately needed" in certain situations. In summary, it appears that the insecticidal approach, which was pioneered by the Rockefeller philanthropies, will be with us into the foreseeable

---

[1] Kim Larsen, Bad Blood, *OnEarth Magazine* 29, Winter 2008, 28.

future, and we ought to have a better idea of how malaria control became hostage to DDT and other insecticides.

The history of DDT is a story of both vision and contingency. The leaders of the two Rockefeller philanthropies who developed and promoted the insecticidal solution to malaria control, the International Health Board, and its successor, the International Health Division of the Rockefeller Foundation, foresaw a technological solution to malaria control. That solution was shaped by several contingencies, including the cooperation of other institutions and of governments, the exigencies of wartime, and the cumulative knowledge derived from fields other than public health, particularly agriculture. This story is of interest in itself — as a tale of epic struggle against disease — but it is also informative as to how we as a global civilization could have gotten to the point of self-contradiction regarding DDT, a "Jekyll and Hyde" chemical that in the early years of the 21st century many people assumed had been consigned to the dustbin of history.

Because of what follows is at its core a history of technology, it will be useful to frame the discussion with a definition of the technologies in question, and particularly how, to a large degree, this particular aspect of the history of malaria has remained outside of the histories of malaria in the 20th century, which have emphasized science and medicine. In fact, two industrial products — Paris Green and DDT — mass-produced chemicals that were developed not to control disease, but first for commercial uses, and later adapted to malaria control, are central to this story. When mixed with various diluents, these are the "technological solutions" that are referred to in the title of this chapter. Secondly, this is a story of the adaptation of hardware that, again, was not contrived for the control of human diseases, but that became vital to the insecticidal approach. Thirdly, this is a story of the triumph of organization of people and the organization of knowledge. The organization of people is for most innovations — as historians of technology often remind us — at least as important as the tools that they use. It may seem somewhat alien to the history of malaria control in the 20th century — which tends to be framed in the epic "microbe hunters" fashion — to discuss such mundane matters as relatively simple chemicals, sprayers, and labor; but it is a premise of this chapter that they are core elements of that history.[2]

My remarks also focus on anti-malaria programs of the International Health Board, created in 1913 (and from 1913 to 1916 officially the International Health Commission), and its direct successor, the International Health Division of the Rockefeller Foundation, as it was styled beginning in 1928. The systematic public

---

[2]The term "microbe hunters" refers to Paul de Kruif's famous book that, among others, focused on the malaria disease discovery work of Ross and Grassi, but not on any anti-malaria projects: Paul de Kruif, *Microbe Hunters*, Harcourt and Brace & Company, 1926: New York.

health work of the Rockefeller philanthropies began with the establishment of the Rockefeller Sanitary Commission for the Eradication of Hookworm Disease in 1909, with a focus on the American South, and quickly evolved into a global public health program carried out by these two entities.[3]

Although malaria certainly was well-known in the American South, the experience of the hookworm program must have brought to the attention of the officers of the Rockefeller Sanitary Commission that many southerners were suffering from multiple diseases and deficiencies, and that malaria probably was chief among them.[4] Moreover, like hookworm disease, both the etiology of the disease and means of controlling it were recent accretions to knowledge, and a frontal assault on the disease seemed possible. One of the first programmatic statements of the International Health Board noted that:

> It has been suggested that some attention should be given to Malaria in the United States and it has been intimated, possibly by Dr. [William] Welch, that this subject is hardly second in importance to that of Hookworm….it may be worthy of consideration whether within a year or two this organization may not be employed in dealing with Malaria….[5]

It was thus in a timely manner that in 1915, Wickliffe Rose presented to the directors of the International Health Board a "Memorandum on Malaria and its Control" that provided both a rationale and a methodology for an anti-malaria program.[6] Strikingly, Rose began by stating that "malarial fevers" were "most prevalent in the tropics where they have proven to be the greatest single obstacle to colonization by the white race."[7] Though my chapter will not examine this premise further, it seems clear enough from this statement that the anti-malaria program was conceived as part of the imperial project of the Western world. Rockefeller public health projects certainly

---

[3] John Ettling, *The Germ of Laziness: Rockefeller Philanthropy and Public Health in the New South*, Harvard University Press, 1981: Cambridge, MA; John Farley, *To Cast Out Disease: A History of the International Health Division of the Rockefeller Foundation (1913-1951)*, Oxford University Press, 2004, 27-31: New York.

[4] An official of the Florida State Board of Health was quoted approvingly as stating that "hookworm disease and malaria should be thought of together as the most serious factor in retarding the mental and physical development of school children and as the greatest handicap to civilization in tropical and subtropical countries.": Memorandum on Malaria and its Control, 2 October 1915, Documents of Record (bound volume), International Health Commission/International Health Board, Rockefeller Foundation Archives (hereafter RFA), Rockefeller Archive Center (hereafter RAC), Sleepy Hollow, New York.

[5] Memo on Rockefeller Foundation, 12 August 1913, folder 123, box 11, RG 3.1, RFA. Thanks to Bethany Antos at the Rockefeller Archive Center for locating this document for me.

[6] Memorandum on Malaria, *op.cit.*

[7] Memorandum on Malaria, *op.cit*, 1.

drew on a world-view that human progress was measured by the advance and triumph of Western civilization. The horrendous prosecution of World War I by the European powers, and eventually by the United States, did little to dim this viewpoint.

Rose's report went on to identify the loci of endemic malaria throughout the world, beginning with North America. He emphasized that portions of the American south were "badly infected" with malaria, and that it was:

> especially common along the southern portion of [the] Mississippi and its tributaries, where certain areas of the [Yazoo] delta are uninhabitable because of the prevalence of this deadly infection.[8]

This observation gave credence to an estimate by Dr. L.C. Howard of the United States Department of Agriculture that there were "no less than 3,000,000 cases of malaria annually," with the result that the annual cost to the United States of unchecked malaria was $100,000,000.[9]

Rose's report then hypothesized that:

> Malaria is a controllable disease. The control measures are determined by the life cycle of the malaria parasite and so far as theory is concerned are definite and simple.[10]

Rose's assertion was unwarranted: malaria had been controlled recently in Havana, Cuba, and in the Panama Canal Zone through heroic measures, but it was unknown whether the control measures applied there might be applicable elsewhere, nor was the critical matter of the life-cycle of the malaria parasite known with confidence. Nonetheless, Rose's view was not only his own but of the Rockefeller "barons," as historian John Farley has labeled them: they frankly believed that American know-how and philanthropy could solve a range of the world's ills.[11]

Rose then argued that malaria control could be carried out through three steps. First, by "the systematic use of quinine," citing the opinion of "[Robert] Koch and his followers [who] insist that it is practicable to eradicate malaria by quinine alone." In other places Rose and others referred to the use of quinine for "sterilizing the blood."[12] At one point there was even reference to "[malaria] control by immunizing

---

[8]Memorandum on Malaria, *op.cit.*, 2.

[9]Memorandum on Malaria, *op.cit.*, 21.

[10]Memorandum on Malaria, *op.cit.*, 35.

[11]Farley, *To Cast Out Disease*, *op.cit.*, 6–20.

[12]E.g., Edwin R. Embree and Wickliffe Rose, No. 7415, Memorandum of Observations of Malaria Control Work about Ruleville in Sunflower County, Mississippi, December 1918, folder 82a, box 15, RG 5.2, RFA; Rockefeller Foundation, *Annual Report for 1918*, 1919, 197: New York.

with quinine," as if quinine were a vaccine.[13] Second, "by protecting man from the bites of the mosquito," which — in a very modern-sounding statement — Rose said could be done through screening houses; using mosquito bed-nets and mosquito repellants; and clearing mosquito habitats around residences.[14]

Finally, Rose turned to "control by mosquito reduction," which he explained at great length, and justified by stating that "if the mosquitoes which convey it be destroyed, the malaria cannot spread, and the parasite having its life cycle broken will be eradicated."[15] Rose then emphasized the success of William Gorgas in controlling yellow fever in the Panama Canal Zone by a bundle of mosquito-reduction methods, and noted that "by employing a combination of measures and by adjusting the emphasis to the needs of the community in question, a greater degree of control under average conditions can be achieved than would be possible by the use of any one measure alone."[16]

Rose's recommendations also followed the strategy of the earlier hookworm campaign by advocating the creation of demonstration projects "to determine the most effective methods of operation; and to standardize the working unit of organization and the cost." He recommended that at least one site should try a quinine-only approach, and that at least one other site should combine quinine administration with measures that would reduce mosquito populations or keep them from easy contact with humans.[17]

When the International Health Commission's board adopted Rose's report on October 26, 1915, Rose was ready to implement it immediately. He had already been in discussions with an officer of the state of Mississippi's board of health, and had agreed that the Yazoo delta area would be one of the trial sites.[18] Subsequently he was sent petitions from officials in Bolivar County, Mississippi who were willing to provide matching funds for anti-malaria work, showing that they were aware of the usual financial precondition in Rockefeller public health campaigns.[19]

---

[13] Rockefeller Foundation, *Annual Report for 1918, op.cit.*, 194.

[14] Memorandum on Malaria, *op.cit.*, 40–1. Rose used the term "mosquito bars for beds" instead of "bed nets."

[15] Memorandum on Malaria, *op.cit.*, 42–3.

[16] Memorandum on Malaria, *op.cit.*, 46.

[17] Memorandum on Malaria, *op.cit.*, 49–50.

[18] Wickliffe Rose to W.S. Leathers, 7 June 1915, folder 37, box 2, RG 5.1.2, RFA; Wickliffe Rose to W.S. Leathers, 10 August 1915, folder 38, box 3, RG 5.1.2, RFA. For an excellent overview of malaria history in the United States, necessarily focused on the southern states, see: Margaret Humphreys, *Malaria: Poverty, Race and Public Health in the United States*, Johns Hopkins University Press, 2001: Baltimore.

[19] W.S. Leathers to Wickliffe Rose, 24 August 1915, with attachment of 17 August 1915, folder 38, box 3, RG 5.1.2, RFA; and W.S. Leathers to Wickliffe Rose, 3 September 1915, folder 38, box 3, RG 5.1.2, RFA; Raymond B. Fosdick, *The Story of the Rockefeller Foundation*, Harper and Brothers, 1952, 35: New York.

Beginning in 1916 all residents of selected communities in Bolivar County were first studied for malaria incidence, then given quinine systematically. After the first year it was reported optimistically that "the degree of malaria control is estimated at 70%."[20] However, there was, at the same time, a growing realization that "greater care [was required] in advising people" so that "a larger percentage of people [will] take quinine in exact accordance with directions."[21] But the Rockefeller officers were discovering that a malaria campaign based on consistent administration of a drug, both in timing and in dosage, could not be sustained. As Margaret Humphreys has pointed out, the quininization campaign foundered on the rock of individual decision-making.[22] In the eyes of the Rockefeller public health officials the coup de grâce for the quinine option was a 1925 study that appeared to demonstrate that, even if the usual standards for quinine administration were followed, quinine did not eliminate all malaria parasites from the blood, as had been assumed.[23]

The alternative malaria-control project was carried out in southeast Arkansas, across the Mississippi River from Bolivar County, at Crossett (Ashley County) and Lake Village (Chicot County) beginning in 1916, and subsequently in other towns nearby. In conjunction with the United States Public Health Service and the Arkansas State Board of Health, the International Health Board employed "methods ... exclusively ... directed against the propagation of mosquitoes."[24] The primal nature of this anti-malaria work in Arkansas, though it has been cited, has not been fully appreciated.[25] The Arkansas sites represented two-thirds of the early anti-malaria work: the efforts there were dedicated to mosquito control, although quinine was administered to anyone found infected after examination of blood smears. In Lake Village, the work was described as "directed toward ascertaining the minimum prophylactic measures that will enable a family to live in health in a

---

[20]C.C. Bass, W.S. Leathers and Wickliffe Rose, No. 789, Memorandum on a Demonstration in the Control of Malaria, 11 December 1915, folder 75, box 14, RG 5.2, RFA; (quote) Wickliffe Rose and W.S. Leathers, Summary Statement of some of the results of the experiments in malaria control in Bolivar County, Mississippi, 20 October 1916, folder 84, box 15, RG 5.2.

[21]C.C. Bass, Plan of Work for Malaria Control in Bolivar County, Mississippi, for the year 1917, folder 84, box 15, RG 5.2, RFA.

[22]Margaret Humphreys, *Malaria: Poverty, Race, and Public Health in the United States*, The Johns Hopkins University Press, 2001, 75: Baltimore.

[23]Humphreys, *Malaria, op.cit.*, 77; Rockefeller Foundation, *Annual Report for 1925*, 1926, 173–4: New York; Memorandum on Malaria, *op.cit.*, 36–7, 39, 51.

[24]Crossett, Arkansas, c. 28 June 1917, folder 140, box 12, RG 5.3, RFA.

[25]Humphreys, *Malaria, op.cit.*, 75; Farley, *To Cast Out Disease, op.cit.*, 109.

malarious community, where drainage is impracticable."[26] In Crossett, a "company town" based on lumbering, according to an early report:

> no attention is given to screening, [to] prophylactic quinine, or to the treatment of malaria carriers. Effort in controlling the diseases is based solely on the description of the breeding places of mosquitoes by the use of drainage, oil drips and by stocking streams with small [mosquito-eating] fish.[27]

In reviewing the work in Bolivar County and the two towns in Arkansas after the first year, it was only the work in Crossett that drew the unqualified admiration of Wickliffe Rose, the head of the International Health Board. He wrote that "this piece of work was very impressive and is one which I believe any town of equal size and equal opportunities for drainage can put into operation."[28]

Here we find some of the earliest evidence of the core value of the public health programs of the International Health Board, and later of the International Health Division of the Rockefeller Foundation. Not that medical and scientific interests were not honored and pursued, but it was the practical, instrumental — if you will, technological — strategies to disease control that enthralled Rockefeller leadership. It was not the Bolivar County quininization model that was followed, but rather the Crossett mosquito-control model that became the centerpiece of the Rockefeller approach. By 1919 the official report of the International Health Board gave top rank among all of its programs to its anti-malaria demonstration projects based on mosquito control, and that same year the discussion of quinine administration was decidedly less enthusiastic than that of mosquito control.[29]

There were circumstances that pushed the Rockefeller leadership in a technological direction. Quininization from the beginning presented problems because "it is found difficult to control the population in a given community." The distribution of quinine posed logistical problems, and it was problematic to get the blood smears needed to identify all the infected and successfully treated individuals. People were moving into or out of the Bolivar County, both temporarily and permanently, much more than had been expected for a rural area.[30] As John Farley has noted, the

---

[26]Wickliffe Rose, Experiments in Anti-Malaria Work: Mississippi, Arkansas, Texas, 20 October 1916, folder 75, box 14, RG 5.2, RFA.

[27]Experiments in Anti-Malaria Work, *op.cit.*

[28]Experiments in Anti-Malaria Work, *op.cit.*

[29]Rockefeller Foundation, *Annual Report for 1919*, 1920, 72, 218–27: New York.

[30]Experiments in Anti-Malaria Work, *op.cit.*

International Health Board had the bad luck to select an area associated with heavy migration to the Northern states of the United States during World War I.[31]

But another important external factor was on the horizon. As early as 1915, the International Health Board had received a report of the use of Paris Green as a mosquito larvicide.[32] A powerful broad-spectrum insecticide, Paris Green (a double salt of copper and arsenic: $3CuHAsO_3 + Cu [C_2H_3O_2]$) had been used as in agriculture in the American South at least since the 1880s.[33] In 1921 a United States Public Health Service officer demonstrated that "Paris green serves as a most effective and inexpensive larvicide for the *Anopheles* mosquito," as noted in the International Health Board's annual report for 1922.[34] Two years later the Board's report referred to "paris-greening," that insecticide's frequent use on Rockefeller anti-malaria projects having turned the noun-and-modifier into a descriptive verb.[35]

Although quininization continued to have its attractions into the early 1920s, and other malaria-control methods were tried, the turn to Paris Green was quite dramatic. This can be illustrated by the experience of IHB officer Lewis Hackett in Brazil (1916–1923), and when he was reassigned from yellow fever work in Brazil to initiate an anti-malaria project in Italy.[36] When the IHB turned its attentions to yellow fever in Brazil in 1922, it was already convinced that mosquito larviciding was the way to go, and even dismissed the Brazilian emphasis on adult mosquito-killing as comparatively wasteful.

Thus when Hackett left Brazil, he was attuned to the IHB's growing focus on anti-larval methods. He was given a tour of the IHB's programs in the American South and saw the early development of Paris Green as a major anti-malaria tool.[37] He became a convert, and during his first two years in Italy developed specific

---

[31] Farley, *To Cast Out Disease, op.cit.*, 110.

[32] W.S. Leathers to John A. Ferrell, 18 September 1915, folder 38, box 3, RG 5.1.2, RFA. Paul Russell states that "The first record of the use of Paris green [as a] mosquito larvicide is a note by B.W. Marston, Sr., in the *New Orleans Times Picayune* of 16 February 1916": Paul Russell, *Man's Mastery of Malaria*, Oxford University Press, 1955, 138: London.

[33] R.H. Loughridge, Report on the Cotton Production in the State of Arkansas, with a Discussion of the General Agricultural Features of the State, in Eugene W. Hilgard, *Report on Cotton Production in the United States. Part I: Mississippi Valley and Southeastern States*, Government Printing Office, 1884, 103: Washington.

[34] Rockefeller Foundation, *Annual Report for 1922*, 1923, 206: New York.

[35] Rockefeller Foundation, *Annual Report for 1924*, 1925, 37: New York.

[36] The following remarks on Lewis Hackett, Brazil and Italy are based on: D.H. Stapleton, Lewis Hackett and the early years of the International Health Board's Yellow Fever Program in Brazil, 1917–1924, *Parassitologia*, 2005, **47**, 353–60.

[37] My remarks on Lewis Hackett in Italy are drawn from: Darwin H. Stapleton, A success for science or technology? The Rockefeller Foundation's role in malaria eradication in Italy, 1924–1935, *Medicina nei Secoli: Arte e Scienza*, 1994, **6**, 213–28.

techniques for utilizing Paris Green in malarious environments there. His Italian colleague, Alberto Missiroli, recalled later that "the discovery of the larvicidal efficiency of Paris Green … led us back with enthusiasm to antilarval methods."[38]

Hackett was vociferous in his opposition to Italy's long-standing national quinine distribution program. He believed that it did nothing to quell malaria and was a waste of money. He also had no appreciation for Italy's program of bonification — manipulating watercourses so that they would silt-in marshy areas, eliminate prime mosquito-breeding areas and convert them into farmland. In both cases, Hackett saw these approaches as accepting the inevitability of malaria, and as allocating resources to projects that, while they might be efficacious in the long-run, were unacceptable diversions from the immediate possibilities of new methods of malaria control.

With Missiroli, Hackett created a model of malaria control based on careful study of each local environment, of the habits of the *Anopheles* species that was the malaria transmitter, of the possibilities for eliminating mosquito-larva habitat, of the distribution of the larva-eating *Gambusia* minnows, and (most importantly) of the use of Paris Green to kill mosquito larva. Although he studied quininization, and tried out various anti-malaria strategies (going so far as to making a trial of the x-raying of spleens), Hackett quickly became a champion of the insecticidal approach.

Importantly, Hackett's and Missiroli's demonstration projects in Italy — under the auspices of their Statione Sperimentale per la Lotta Anti-Malarica in Rome — became the focus of the International Health Board's anti-malaria work during the decade of the Stazione's operation (1925–1935). Malariologists and public health workers from around the world were sent to the Stazione to learn the insecticidal approach. The Foundation's published annual reports emphasized its effectiveness. In 1929, for example, there was an effusive statement about the Hackett-Missiroli project at Fiumicino, where Rome's international airport is now located. It is worth quoting the statement at some length:

> The town of Fiumicino, Italy, and the adjacent areas of Ostia on the south and Maccarese on the north, constitute one of the impressive demonstrations in Europe of the effect of antilarval work on malaria incidence… Classical methods of malaria control — major drainage and the use of quinine — had been tried for a long time. In 1926 the central Malaria Station at Rome took over the work at Fiumicino, and malaria at once fell to a new low level which has been further decreased each succeeding year. Only when the mosquito density was brought down to a certain

---

[38] Alberto Missiroli, *Anopheles* control in the Mediterranean area, *Proceedings of the Fourth International Congresses on Tropical Medicine and Malaria*, Government Printing Office, 1948, **2**, 1566: Washington.

level did malaria start its final descent to the vanishing point. Here, then, is a picture of three typical areas in which major drainage, prophylactic quinine, and intensive treatment over a period of thirty years failed to cause any significant diminution in malaria ... [but] three years of sustained attack on anopheline breeding has made malaria a sporadic and rare infection.[39]

Through visits to the Italian project hosted by Hackett and Missiroli, a global cohort of malariologists was introduced to the insecticidal approach: these included representatives from Brazil, Britain, France, Netherlands, Soviet Union, and Sri Lanka, as well as the League of Nations Malaria Commission.[40] Hackett also promoted his techniques through his book *Malaria in Europe* (1937), which became a fundamental text for many of his generation.

Hackett's program in Italy was closed down in 1935 when the Istituto di Sanità Pubblica — the Rockefeller-funded institute of public health for Italy — was fully in operation.[41] He continued to oversee various anti-malaria projects in southern Europe, but his work was no longer the most innovative in the Rockefeller sphere. That mantle passed to Paul Russell and his little-remarked work in India from 1936 to 1942.

Russell previously had been involved with the International Health Board's anti-malaria work in the American South, and then in Singapore and the Philippines. In India, he carried out several demonstration projects intended to persuade local governments to undertake anti-malaria work (which the British colonial government was reluctant to fund) by showing them how cheaply it could be done. A critical complement to Russell was provided when in 1938 engineer Fred Knipe was assigned to serve under him, fresh from collaborations with Lewis Hackett, which had included Paris-greening work. Russell and Knipe carried out not only larvicidal projects with Paris Green, but also tests with pyrethrum, a powerful insecticide derived from chrysanthemum flowers, to kill adult mosquitoes resting in buildings. In the test town of Kasangadu it was reported that the spleen index, a standard measurement of malaria infection, dropped from 68% to 5% in three years of spraying.[42]

---

[39] Rockefeller Foundation, *Annual Report for 1929*, 1930, 75: New York.

[40] Darwin H. Stapleton, Fellowships and Field Stations: the Globalization of Public Health Knowledge, 1920–1950, presented at the Joint Learning Initiative, History Working Group, Bellagio Conference Center, October 2003 (unpublished).

[41] Gianfranco Donelli and Enrica Serinaldi, *Dalla Lotta alla Malaria alla Nascita Dell'Istituto di Sanità Pubblica: Il Ruolo della Rockefeller Foundation in Italia: 1922–1934*, Editori Laterza, 2003, 214: Rome. The Istituto di Sanità Pubblica became the Istituto Superiore di Sanita after World War II.

[42] D.H. Stapleton, Technology and malaria control, 1930–1960: the career of Rockefeller Foundation engineer Frederick W. Knipe, *Parassitologia*, 2000, **42**, 59–68.

Paul Russell and Frederick Knipe gained important insights into malaria control during their years in India, and influenced the malaria program of the Rockefeller Foundation in ways that are not yet fully appreciated.[43] But it certainly seems more than coincidental that the Foundation's approach to anti-mosquito work shifted from an almost purely larvicidal approach to one that included using sprays to kill adult mosquitoes. Unfortunately, with the entrance of the United States into World War II, Russell and Knipe were withdrawn from India and their experimental work was stopped; but they became leaders in malaria control after the war, drawing on their experience in India.[44]

The next wave of innovation came unexpectedly from Switzerland, where Paul Müller, with the Geigy chemical firm, discovered in 1939 that a long-known chemical, now called DDT ($CCl_3CH[C_6H_4Cl]_2$), was an incredibly effective insecticide. To cut the story short, Geigy made samples of DDT available to American, British and German agencies in the latter half of 1942, and the United States began manufacturing it in the spring of 1943.[45]

The Rockefeller Foundation carried out the most important of the field tests of DDT — on the American side — during the war. At first the Foundation focused on DDT as an anti-typhus measure in North Africa during the summer of 1943, because it was anticipated that typhus could be rampant when the Allies invaded Europe. The Rockefeller tests showed emphatically the power of DDT, and when there was an apparent typhus epidemic in Naples in late 1943 after the Allies took control of Sicily and lower Italy, DDT proved to be effective in stopping it. Thereafter DDT "marched with the troops" throughout Europe.[46]

DDT was quickly turned to the fight against other insect-borne diseases: in the Pacific, DDT was sprayed on beaches and islands even before the Allied forces landed to fight malaria and dengue fever; and before the end of the war,

---

[43] For a document that connects Russell's India campaign with his later involvement with DDT see: Paul Russell to Fred Soper, 1 November 1948, folder 463, box 48, series 100I, RG 1.1, RFA.

[44] Darwin H. Stapleton, Lessons of history? Anti-malaria strategies of the International Health Board and the Rockefeller Foundation from the 1920s to the era of DDT, *Public Health Reports*, March-April 2004, **119**, 209–10.

[45] On the early testing of DDT for its possible effects on human health, see: Edmund P. Russell III, The strange career of DDT: experts, federal capacity, and environmentalism in World War II, *Technology and Culture*, 1999, **40**, 770–98.

[46] Darwin H. Stapleton, A lost chapter in the history of DDT: the development of anti-typhus technologies by the Rockefeller Foundation's Louse Laboratory, 1942–1944, *Technology and Culture*, July 2005, **46**, 513–40; Darwin H. Stapleton, The Short-lived miracle of DDT, *American Heritage of Invention and Technology*, Winter 2000, **15**, 34–41; Darwin H. Stapleton, DDT Marches with the Troops in North Africa and Italy: Developing an Insecticide Technology as a Tool of War, 1943–45, read at the 27th Symposium of the International Committee for the History of Technology, Prague, Czech Republic, 22–26 August 2000 (unpublished).

Rockefeller officers began testing DDT as an anti-malaria insecticide in Italy. In both cases the efforts were aimed at killing adult insects, not flies or mosquitoes in larval stages.

This work set the stage for the Foundation's most famous effort, the five-year attempt to eradicate all malaria-carrying mosquitoes from Sardinia, carried out with the approval of the Italian government and largely funded by the United Nations Relief and Rehabilitation Administration. Although based on the spraying of DDT, both by teams of *disinfestores* who attempted to reach every nook and cranny of the island, and by broad-swath aerial spraying, we should understand that the Sardinian project was focused as much on the organization of manpower, as it was on DDT. It also drew on Fred Knipe's experience with individual sprayers, and provided a platform for him to try to develop the simplest, lowest-cost DDT sprayer possible.[47] The Sardinian project, like the work in Italy two decades earlier, was exploited by the Rockefeller Foundation as a demonstration project: dozens of public health leaders from around the globe came to Sardinia to observe and to learn. Since many of those leaders had been Foundation or International Health Board fellows who had been previously inculcated with the Rockefeller technological strategy for malaria control, they were primed to accept the lesson, and went back to their home countries enthralled with the prospects that DDT held. The massive publicity (including widely-distributed films) accompanying the Sardinian project has tended to obscure other Foundation's other DDT projects of significance, such as those in Mexico, and Trinidad and Tobago.[48]

The Foundation's DDT tests in Mexico, beginning in the spring of 1945, were carried out at the behest of the United States Department of Agriculture's Bureau of Entomology and Plant Quarantine. In spite of what was reported as "a healthy skepticism" by the Mexican Ministry of Health, the Foundation (which had a twenty-year history of public health work in Mexico) pursued DDT testing in the state of Morelos. The project focused exclusively on spraying DDT on the walls of dwellings, for the purpose of killing adult mosquitoes. Two months after the start of spraying, there was a 99% reduction in the incidence of *Anopheles* mosquitoes in the dwellings. This demonstration was so impressive that the next year the Mexican government asked for an expansion of DDT spraying, so that in 1947 the Foundation's program was expanded to the state of Veracruz and the next year to the states of Chiapas and Baja California, and to a portion of the Federal

---

[47]Stapleton, Technology and malaria control, *op.cit.*, 65–6.
[48]Two major films were "Adventure in Sardinia" (1948), and "The Sardinian Project" (1949). See: Marianne Fedunkiw, Malaria films: motion pictures as a public health tool, *American Journal of Public Health*, July 2003, **93**, 1046–57.

District. From that point the Mexican government and later the United States's Point IV program became involved in DDT spraying on a large scale, and the Foundation's efforts were phased out by 1952.[49] Nonetheless, the Foundation's work had launched Mexico on one of the most extensive anti-malaria projects undertaken in the world.[50]

The Foundation began anti-malaria work in Trinidad and Tobago after the United States took over British military bases there early in 1941.[51] Soon after an officer of the United States Army Medical Corps recommended that the Rockefeller Foundation undertake a survey of malaria conditions there, arguing that "the Rockefeller organization is the best qualified health agency in the world to conduct this survey."[52] Foundation officers arrived in 1942 and began anti-malaria work of the classic type, including identifying the habits of the *Anopheles* vector, improving drainage, and destruction of mosquito habitat. The Trinidad and Tobago project had many visitors, becoming a wartime training site for malariologists from the Caribbean and Latin America.[53]

In the fall of 1944 the first quantity of DDT arrived in Trinidad for testing, although Rockefeller staff there had long known about its impressive qualities. Raymond Shannon, the entomologist on the staff at Trinidad and Tobago, soon wrote to the head of the International Health Division that "the introduction of DDT necessitates a revision of practically our entire program of field investigations," and that the aerial spraying of DDT would allow the reaching of "the major anopheline breeding areas [which were] ... practically impassable" for vehicles, and that "it would not be feasible to attempt extensive use of DDT as a larvicide by manpower."[54] He recommended selecting the island of Tobago for an attempt at permanent eradication of malaria-carrying mosquitoes.

---

[49] D.H. Stapleton, The dawn of DDT and its experimental use by the Rockefeller Foundation in Mexico, 1943–1952, *Parassitologia*, 1998, **40**, 149–58.

[50] H. Gómez-Dantés and A.E. Birn, Malaria and social movements in Mexico: the last 60 years, *Parassitologia*, 2000, **42**, 73–80.

[51] For a view of the United States's acquisition of a military base in Trinidad see: http://www.triniview.com/Carenage-Chaguaramas/Chaguaramas2.html. Site viewed on 20 October 2008.

[52] Leon A. Fox, Sanitary Survey of Trinidad, B.W.I., June 1941, folder 35, box 3, series 451, RG 1.1, RFA.

[53] Darwin H. Stapleton, The Rockefeller Foundation's Experimental Strategies for Using DDT to Control Malaria in the Caribbean Region, 1943–1951: The Case of Trinidad and Tobago (presented at the conference), The Social History of Medicine and Public Health in the Caribbean, University of the West Indies, Cave Hill Campus, Barbados, 23–26 May 2001 (unpublished).

[54] R.C. Shannon to G.K. Strode, Reply to Dr. Strode's Memorandum Dealing with Malaria Investigations, November 29, 1944, folder 39, box 3, series 451, RG 1.1, RFA.

Shannon's eradication idea was recommended to the International Health Division's Board of Scientific Directors in March 1946, and the next year the Division approved of the saturation DDT spraying of Tobago, noting that:

> With the development of new drugs and insecticides, it has become possible to think of complete eradication of malaria and anophelines in various parts of the world. Tobago, because of its small size, seems especially suitable for such a campaign in the Western Hemisphere.[55]

The Foundation's president, Raymond Fosdick, offered a similar, but more expansive, sentiment a year later in his annual review when he offered a science-fiction tinged view of the future:

> We seem to be on the threshold of an era more promising than any we have known. The sulfonamides, penicillin, radioactive isotopes, DDT ... foreshadow a new move forward, a new renaissance, a new period in human development when the imagination is endowed with wings.[56]

DDT was mesmerizing: it held the power to herald "a new period in human development."

Although the Foundation funded, but did not directly oversee the Tobago operation, it followed the project closely. Only eighteen months into the program it was reported that "malaria transmission has been reduced practically to zero" on the island, and by the summer of 1950 there were almost no anophelines to be found on Tobago.

Considering that the Foundation had a mosquito-eradication program in Sardinia, as well as funded or closely-watched DDT-spraying programs on the islands of Cyprus, Sri Lanka, and Taiwan, one could say that in the postwar era, the Foundation had embarked on an "island program" of DDT demonstration projects at globally-strategic sites.[57] At each of these sites, as well as the other countries where the Foundation was involved in anti-malaria work, the broader visions of malariologists were downplayed or ignored; the Foundation's new approach appeared to strip away the need to understand the entomological,

---

[55]Estimates — 1948 — Malaria, Tobago — Malaria and *Anopheline* Control, $17,200, 31 October 1947, folder 37, box 3, series 451, RG 1.1, RFA.

[56]Rockefeller Foundation, *Annual Report for 1947*, 1948, 25: New York.

[57]Department of Health, Republic of China, Malaria Eradication in Taiwan, 1991, 17–33; K. Constantinou, *Anopheles* (malaria) eradication in Cyprus, *Parassitologia*, 1998, **40**, 131–5; K. Yip, Malaria eradication: the Taiwan experience, *Parassitologia*, 2000, **42**, 119–21.

environmental and social parameters of malaria. In 1948, one Mexican public health officer, for example, told a Rockefeller Foundation officer that it now appeared that "no malariologists, engineers, or entomologists are now necessary" for an anti-malaria campaign.[58] The use of DDT; the techniques of spraying (primarily to kill adult mosquitoes); and the organization of labor such that the spraying could be done systematically and cheaply, were now the focus of the anti-malaria campaigns. What I have related provides underpinning for Randall Packard's conclusion in his recent masterful work *The Making of a Tropical Disease: A Short History of Malaria.*[59] In his words:

> [E]fforts to control malaria since the end of the nineteenth century have been largely driven by a [narrow] vision of the disease and its causes that has privileged biological processes and focused on attacking anopheline mosquitoes and malaria parasites.[60]

This "narrow vision" was framed in large part by the Rockefeller fascination with technological solutions, created by the mid-twentieth century a global revolution in anti-malaria strategies, a revolution that we are continuing to cope with today.[61]

---

[58] Hugh H. Smith diary entry, 26 March–4 April 1948, folder 151, box 18, series 323I, RG 1.1, RFA.

[59] Randall M. Packard, *The Making of a Tropical Disease: A Short History of Malaria*, Johns Hopkins University Press, 2007: Baltimore.

[60] Packard, *The Making of a Tropical Disease*, op.cit., 247.

[61] Brenda Eskenazi, *et al.*, eds.,The Pine River statement: human health consequences of DDT use, *Environmental Health Perspectives*, September 2009, **117**, 1359–67. This paper resulted from the "Eugene Kenaga International DDT Conference on Environment and Health" at Alma College (Alma, MI) in March 2008.

3 Malaria Control and Eradication Projects in Tropical Africa, 1945–1965

James L.A. Webb, Jr.

"…the controversy as to whether or not control of malaria is of ultimate benefit to the African… is without doubt the most urgent problem requiring investigation and until an answer can be given malaria control is not on sure foundations nor can a policy be defined."

— Malaria Sub-Committee of the Colonial
Medical Research Committee (U.K.), 1946.[1]

The global burden of malaria today is centered on tropical Africa.[2] The high levels of year-round malaria transmission, the high mosquito vector densities, and the low levels of African incomes — which limit the abilities of African communities to protect themselves from malaria — present intractable difficulties for disease control. The contemporary campaigns to control and 'eliminate' malaria are based principally upon a program of vector control using insecticide-treated bednets and indoor residual spraying (IRS) of insecticides in an effort to reduce transmission, and secondarily upon chemical therapy using the new generation of artemisisin-based antimalarial drugs.[3] This campaign has scored some successes in reducing

---

[1]Malaria Sub-Committee of the Colonial Medical Research Committee, 1946, CMR (ML) (46) 9, piece 24, page 1, CO 913/14, National Archives of the United Kingdom.

[2]An earlier version of this paper was presented at the 2008 Yale conference on the Global Crisis of Malaria. I would like to thank Prof. Frank Snowden for the invitation to address the conference, and for his innovative initiative in bringing historians and malaria scientists together. I conducted archival research for this essay at the World Health Organization in Geneva, Switzerland. I wish to acknowledge with gratitude the kind assistance of the WHO archivist, Mme. Marie Villemin Partow. The Social Science Research Committee of Colby College provided travel funds that made this archival research possible.

[3]For a contemporary prospectus for global malaria eradication, see Richard G.A. Feachem, Allison A. Phillips, and Geoffrey A. Targett (eds.), *Shrinking the Malaria Map: A Prospectus on Malaria Elimination*, The Global Health Group, 2009: San Francisco, CA.

the levels of morbidity and mortality in tropical Africa, although the number of childhood deaths remains very high.[4]

Introduction

This chapter explores the early efforts at malaria control and eradication in tropical Africa in the period 1945–1965. It discusses the attempts to transfer and adapt techniques and knowledge about malaria control that had been gained elsewhere to the African tropics. The World Health Organization (WHO) provided technical assistance to some of the pilot projects that attempted to determine the practicality of fully interrupting the transmission of malaria through the use of synthetic insecticides alone or, when this proved unachievable, in combination with the administration of antimalarial drugs to the African populations in the project zones. At length, the researchers uncovered what seemed to be intractable biophysical and cultural realities about malaria transmission in Africa.

A Basis For Optimism, I — Malaria Control Outside of Tropical Africa

In the aftermath of World War II, the technical prospects for the control of malaria appeared promising. The success of antimalaria interventions in war-ravaged Italy, in the southern states of the U.S.A., and in Mexico — in zones of mixed *vivax*, *malariae*, and *falciparum* infections — encouraged malariologists to expand their use of synthetic insecticides to other malarious areas.[5] Dichloro-diphenyl-trichloroethane (DDT), in particular, promised an inexpensive method of vector control, and raised the prospect of effective public health interventions without having to create public health systems. At the time, this seemed to be the essence of public health economy. Enthusiasms ran high. In the immediate postwar period, malaria control campaigns were launched in Greece, Corsica, Venezuela, and Ceylon. In 1946, the first-ever campaign of malaria eradication began on the island of Sardinia. Its strategic goal was to test the feasibility of using DDT to rid the island of its malarial vector, *Anopheles labranchiae*, and thus malaria itself, the island's principal disease burden.[6]

---

[4]Robert W. Snow and Kevin Marsh, Malaria in Africa: progress and prospects in the decade since the Abuja Declaration, *The Lancet,* 10 July 2010, **376**, 137–9.

[5]On the Italian experience, see Frank M. Snowden, *The Conquest of Malaria: Italy, 1900–1962,* Yale University Press, 2006, 181–97: New Haven, CT; on the U.S. experience, Margaret Humphreys, Kicking a dying dog: DDT and the demise of malaria in the American South, *Isis,* 1996, **87**, no. 1, 1–17; on the Mexican experience, Darwin H. Stapleton, The dawn of DDT and its experimental use by the Rockefeller Foundation in Mexico, 1943–1952, *Parassitologia,* 1998, **40**, 149–58.

[6]Gordon Harrison, *Mosquitoes, Malaria, and Man: A History of the Hostilities Since 1880,* E.P. Dutton, 1978, 223–4: New York. On the changing goals of the Sardinian campaign, see

Some malariologists were cautious about the prospects in tropical Africa. They understood that the African malaria problem was different and more severe. The two principal African mosquito vectors — *Anopheles funestus, Anopheles gambiae sensu stricto*, and *Anopheles arabiensis* (once considered part of an *Anopheles gambiae* complex) — were highly efficient; and *Anopheles funestus* and *Anopheles gambiae sensu stricto* took most of their blood meals from human beings, rather than from domesticated livestock or animals in the wild. They maintained high levels of endemic malarial infection. Moreover, the large majority of Africans (in West and West Central Africa as much as 97 percent or so of the populations) carried a hemoglobin mutation that protected against the more common and less virulent globally distributed *vivax* malaria parasite. This meant that most malaria infections in tropical Africa were caused by the *falciparum* parasite that produced the most deadly form of the disease.[7]

Yet there were grounds for optimism. Malariologists had rung up two major successes in species eradication against an African vector, albeit outside of its endemic environments. In late 1929 or early 1930, an African mosquito traveled aboard a fast French destroyer carrying mail across the Atlantic from Dakar to northeastern Brazil and triggered a malaria epidemic there.[8] Fred L. Soper and D. Bruce Wilson of the Rockefeller Foundation countered the anopheline invasion. They imposed a military-style discipline on the Brazilian antimalaria teams, who achieved 'species eradication" through extensive larviciding and housespraying, eliminating the African vector from Brazil; the disease itself, however, continued to be transmitted by the less-efficient indigenous anopheline mosquitoes.[9] (In 2008, molecular investigations revealed that the African vector introduced to Brazil was in fact *Anopheles arabiensis*, not *Anopheles gambiae* as it had been long held.)[10]

During the Second World War, malariologists scored the second important victory. In the early 1940s, *Anopheles gambiae*, introduced from below the Sahara, ignited a malarial conflagration in Egypt that resulted in the deaths of between one and two hundred thousand people. As in Brazil, an aggressive larviciding program — in which Soper played a significant role — successfully disrupted the breeding of *Anopheles gambiae*. By 1945, the Egyptian outbreak had been fully suppressed, and *Anopheles*

Peter J. Brown, Failure as success: multiple meanings of eradication in the Rockefeller Foundation Sardinia Project, *Parassitologia*, 1998, **40**, 117–30.

[7]On the early establishment of malaria in tropical Africa, see James L.A. Webb Jr., *Humanity's Burden: A Global History of Malaria*, Cambridge University Press, 2009, 17–41: New York.

[8]Fred L. Soper and D. Bruce Wilson, *Anopheles Gambiae in Brazil, 1930 to 1940*, The Rockfeller Foundation, 1943, 22–3: New York.

[9]Soper and Wilson, *Anopheles Gambiae, op.cit.*, passim.

[10]Aristides Parmakelis *et al.*, Short Report: historical analysis of a near disaster: *Anopheles Gambiae* in Brazil, *American Journal of Tropical Medicine and Hygiene*, 2008, **78**(1), 176–8.

gambiae had been regionally banished.[11] In both Brazil and Egypt, the malariologists had laid down the chemical larvicide known as Paris Green, whose insecticidal powers had been in the antimalarial arsenal since the 1920s.[12]

Another heartening achievement in malaria control — and near eradication — radiated from British Guiana. There, in 1945, the physician and malariologist George Giglioli launched an IRS program using DDT to control the local vector *Anopheles darlingi*. His approach was so successful that it appeared that it might be possible to eradicate locally an indigenous vector and, perhaps, to prevent its reintroduction.[13] By extension, this suggested the possibility of a broader application for vector control in the South American tropics, if the approach could be 'scaled-up.' It also suggested that DDT might be very effective in another tropical context — on the African side of the South Atlantic.

A Basis for Optimism, II — Malaria Control in Africa Before and Immediately After WWII

In the early 1930s in the subtropics of southern Africa, G.A. Park Ross, a South African malariologist, pioneered the IRS vector control strategy, spraying the walls and ceilings of human habitations with pyrethrum insecticides to kill adult mosquitoes. Pyrethrum insecticides worked well, but their killing powers dissipated quickly. Walls and ceilings had to be resprayed frequently in order to reduce the transmission of malaria, and this was expensive. The early experiences with indoor spraying seemed technically promising, and in 1935 further experiments were called for at the Pan-African Health Conference convened in Johannesburg. The conference committee, however, saw no realistic prospects for large-scale antimalaria intervention in rural Africa that were not linked to economic improvements in the Africans' standards of living.[14]

---

[11] The natural insecticide made from chrysanthemum flowers known as pyrethrum was scarce and expensive, but some was held in reserve for use for IRS in the event that larviciding failed to disrupt the breeding of *Anopheles gambiae*. Weekly IRS with pyrethrum was used with good effect in Upper Egypt in the 18,000 houses in the El Badari region. [Aly Tewfik Shousha, The eradication of *Anopheles Gambiae* from Upper Egypt, 1942–1945, *Bulletin of the World Health Organization*, 1948, 1(2), 309–52; on pyrethrum spraying in El Badari, 326–7.]

[12] The first use of Paris Green was in the 1870s against the Colorado potato beetle. R.A. Casagrande, Colorado Potato Beetle: 125 Years of mismanagement, *Bulletin of the Entomological Society of America*, 1987, 33(3), 144.

[13] G. Giglioli, Malaria control in British Guiana, *Bulletin of the World Health Organization,* 1954, 11, 849–53; George Giglioli, *Demerara Doctor: An Early Success Against Malaria. The Autobiography of a Self-Taught Physician, George Giglioli (1897–1975)*, Smith–Gordon, 2006, 205–18: London.

[14] [n.a.] (Pan-African Health Conference), Malaria under African conditions, *Quarterly Bulletin of the Health Organisation of the League of Nations,* 1936, 5, 110–3; Annex I, G.A. Park Ross,

These early pyrethrum spraying experiences were an important influence on later control efforts within tropical Africa, yet specialists recognized that there were important ecological differences between the broader southern African region and the core regions of tropical Africa: the southern African vectors were dangerous — particularly *Anopheles funestus* — but the region did not have to contend with a heavy presence of *Anopheles gambiae sensu stricto*, a principal vector elsewhere in sub-Saharan Africa; and transmission was seasonal rather than year-round.[15]

The southern African malarial control efforts did share some common aspects with efforts in the African tropics. Most of the malaria control efforts focused on what today would be called "environmental management techniques," the drainage and filling in of mosquito habitat and the use of larvicides on surface waters. The use of quinine as a prophylactic and curative drug was principally reserved to the European community. The goal of the control efforts was to protect the health of the Europeans and the Africans who worked on European farms and plantations and in the mines or who lived in cities and large towns with sizeable European populations. Europeans saw that malarial infections undermined African worker morale and productivity, and where African workers or urban dwellers lived in close proximity to Europeans, the health of the Africans was perceived as directly relevant to the health of the Europeans.

The Transfer of Synthetic Insecticide, 1945–1950

The first large-scale use of synthetic insecticides for IRS below the Sahara began in 1945 in Monrovia, Liberia, and after some initial successes, the malaria program was 'scaled-up' into the region surrounding Monrovia.[16] A small-scale house-spraying program with DDT began in Southern Rhodesia (Zimbabwe) the same year, and in subsequent years programs of IRS using DDT began in several

---

Insecticide as a major measure in the control of malaria, being an account of the methods and organisation put in force in natal and Zululand during the past six years, *Quarterly Bulletin of the Health Organisation of the League of Nations*, 1936, **5**, 114–33; and Annex II, B. De Meillon, The control of malaria in South Africa by measures directed against the adult mosquitoes in habitations, *Quarterly Bulletin of the Health Organisation of the League of Nations,* 1936, **5**, 134–7.

[15] For the distribution of malarial vectors in tropical Africa, see Jean Mouchet *et al.*, *Biodiversité du paludisme dans le monde*, John Libby Eurotext, 2004, 66–75: Paris; for *Anopheles gambiae*: 68 and *Anopheles funestus*: 72.

[16] James L.A. Webb Jr., The first large-scale use of synthetic insecticides to control malaria in tropical Africa: lessons from Liberia, 1945–1962, *Journal of the History of Medicine and Allied Sciences*, 2011, **66**(3), 347–76.

regions of southern Africa, including South Africa, Swaziland, Bechuanaland (Botswana), and southern Mozambique.[17]

These early IRS programs aimed at the control of malarial disease. As these efforts enjoyed success, some of the projects began to focus on localized species eradication. What had worked against invasive species in Brazil and Egypt and against an indigenous species in British Guiana led to hopes for success against indigenous species in tropical Africa.[18]

In the last years of the 1940s, another success in species eradication on the island of Mauritius appeared as a harbinger of future campaigns in the 'war on malaria.' Even before the arrival in 1948 of a small malaria control team dispatched by the Colonial Insecticides Committee (U.K.) to attempt species eradication by residual spraying, efforts at malaria control had reduced malaria transmission to virtually nil in the densely populated residential plateau in the middle of the island and the business district of the capital, Port Louis. And from 1949 to 1951, M.A.C. Dowling, a young British physician, led a team that succeeded in eliminating *Anopheles funestus* from the island, completely inter-rupting malaria transmission, and reducing the population of *Anopheles gambiae* by more than 98 percent. In 1951, Dowling tried to move in for the kill, launching a larvicidal program to eradicate *Anopheles gambiae*. Disappointment ensued. Following heavy rainfall in February 1952, *Anopheles gambiae* increased its reproduction in spite of the eradication teams' best efforts. Hopes for the species eradication of *Anopheles gambiae* were given up, and future malaria control efforts focused on surveillance and treatment of imported cases.[19]

---

[17]Other IRS programs with DDT began in the 1960s in Namibia and Southern Rhodesia (Zimbabwe). Musawenkosi L.H. Mabaso, Brian Sharp, and Christian Lengeler, Historical review of malarial control in Southern Africa with emphasis on the use of indoor residual house-spraying, *Tropical Medicine and International Health*, 2004, **9**(8), 846–56.

An experiment in malaria control was undertaken in Freetown in 1947, with disappointing results. R. Elliott, Use of DDT as a Residual Insecticide for the Control of Malaria in Freetown, 1947, SJ1, JK1, Sierra Leone, WHO 7.0039, World Health Organization Archives, Geneva.

[18]In the view of Fred Soper of the Rockefeller Foundation, who had directed the campaign against *Anopheles arabiensis* in Brazil, a basic principle was the necessity for an attack on a sufficiently large area so that reinfestation from unworked areas could not pose a problem. Fred L. Soper, Species sanitation as applied to the eradication of (A) an invading or (B) an indigenous species, *Proceedings of the Fourth International Congress on Tropical Medicine and Malaria*, United States Government Printing Office, 1948, **1**, 854: Washington, DC.

[19]M.A.C. Dowling, The malaria eradication scheme in Mauritius, *British Medical Bulletin*, 1951, **8**, 72–5; M.A.C. Dowling, Malaria control in Mauritius, *British Medical Bulletin*, 1952, **9**, 339; M.A.C. Dowling, Control of malaria in Mauritius: eradication of *Anopheles funestus* and *Aedes aegypti*, *Transactions of the Royal Society of Tropical Medicine and Hygiene*, 1953, **47**(3), 177–98.

Even as the Mauritius eradication efforts advanced, malariologists on the African mainland launched some experiments to determine the feasibility of using DDT against the anopheline vectors in rural, tropical Africa. The initial results were mixed. In the Kipsigis reserve in western Kenya, 2,500 huts were sprayed with DDT in three cycles in 1946. The experiment reduced deaths in comparison to a control area, and drove down the parasite rate and reduced the vector density.[20] The Belgian Fonds du Bien-Être Indigène in Ruanda-Urundi, in collaboration with the J.R. Geigy S.A., the Swiss manufacturer of DDT, in March 1949 sprayed a small number of huts in the mountains. The team concluded that IRS would be efficacious in reducing the parasite levels of the populations, and then scaled-up the experiment to cover roughly 20,000 to 23,000 people. Teams of insecticide sprayers dosed African huts and anopheline-breeding habitats. Adult mosquito density in the huts declined markedly, but the mosquitoes propagated in their breeding grounds.[21]

The First African Malaria Conference: Kampala, 1950

The WHO and the Commission for Technical Cooperation in Africa South of the Sahara jointly convened a Malaria Conference in Equatorial Africa in Kampala in late 1950. Malariologists from the WHO, many of the European states with colonies in tropical Africa (Great Britain, Portugal, France, and Belgium), Liberia, and the U.S.A. attended. The participants had the benefit of a report by Dr. F.J.C. Cambournac, a professor at the Lisbon Institute of Tropical Medicine and Director of the Institute of Malariology, Agues de Moura, Portugal. He had been charged by the Director-General of the World Health Organization with the preparation of a report on malaria control efforts in equatorial Africa and toward this end, he had traveled for more than six months logging nearly 48,000 miles.[22]

The last indigenous case of malaria occurred in 1965. Leonard J. Bruce-Chwatt, Malaria in Mauritius — as dead as the Dodo, *Bulletin of the New York Academy of Medicine,* November 1974, **50**(10), 1079.

[20] P.C.C. Garnham. DDT versus malaria, Kenya 1946—commentary on a film, in E.E. Sabben-Clare, D.J. Bradley, and K. Kirkwood (eds.), *Health in Tropical Africa During the Colonial Period,* Clarendon Press, 1980, 64–65: Oxford.

[21] Compte-rendu concernant l'activité de la Mission d'étude de désinsectisation envoyée au Ruanda-Urundi par le Fonds du Bien-Etre Indigène en collaboration avec la maison J.R. Geigy S.A. Bâle. Février-août 1949, 44–54 WHO7.0038. JKT 1, SJ1; J. Jaden, A. Fain, and H. Rupp., Lutte anti-malarienne étendue en zone rurale au moyen de D.D.T. à Astrida, Ruanda-Urundi, *Institut Royal Colonial Belge, Section des Sciences Naturelles et Médicales, Mémoires,* 1952, **21**(fasc. 1), 1–47.

[22] Dr. F.J.C. Cambournac, Report on Malaria in Equatorial Africa, WHO/Mal/58.

At the Kampala conference, the major policy issue was whether to undertake IRS campaigns in rural African regions of intense malaria transmission. Africans in these zones who had survived childhood infections acquired immunity to malaria and as a result suffered less severe bouts. Some were heavily parasitized and remained entirely asymptomatic. The maintenance of acquired immunity depended on recurrent inoculations with the malarial parasites. One concern was that the interventions, if successful, might compromise the Africans' acquired malaria immunities, about which little was known. If the control efforts were to subsequently fail, the populations that had been 'protected' by the IRS campaigns might lose their immunities and suffer "rebound" epidemic malaria with serious consequences. A partial counter-argument was that Africans' acquired immunities might well be lost in other processes anyway, such as the movements of rural African laborers to cities, mines, or European-directed plantations. In this view, "economic progress" might involve increases in morbidity and mortality for adults with fully functional acquired immunities whose immunological defenses degraded owing to a reduction in infective inoculations.[23]

During the conference sessions, heated exchanges erupted between experts. The dispute over IRS was contentious because professional opinions differed over whether the high levels of inoculations (and thus the continued challenge by malaria parasites) in regions of heavy endemic transmission produced a fully functional acquired immunity — that is, full protection from malarial sickness in adult populations. Cambournac had put the problem bluntly in his preconference report: "… control measures partially carried out or continued for a limited time are dangerous, since the populations of formerly hyperendemic regions will obviously be exposed to the risk of severe epidemics, involving serious consequences."[24] If so, partial or time-limited interventions that caused the loss of acquired immunity might well produce sickness and perhaps even deaths in the formerly immune populations.

Two camps formed. One favored malaria intervention using IRS in rural areas and the other favored a more cautious investigation of the consequences of the interruption of acquired immunity. The dominant faction at the Kampala conference endorsed a policy proposal to move forward with malaria control as soon as it was feasible, whatever the degree of endemic malaria. To address the concerns of the experts on the potential consequences of the loss of fully functional immunities, they advised that the regions with the higher levels of endemic infection would require the establishment of an effective malaria control organization that would be able to intervene with insecticides and drugs, should epidemic malaria erupt after the ending of the control projects. (This would be largely honored in

[23]Report of the Malaria Conference in Equatorial Africa, WHO/Mal/69, 22.
[24]Dr. F.J.C. Cambournac, Report on Malaria in Equatorial Africa, WHO/Mal/58, 66.

the breach.) And they recommended that the WHO advise on the malaria control projects in one or more areas in which the populations appeared to have a high degree of tolerance.[25]

The core empirical questions were yet to be answered: Would it be possible to interrupt the transmission of malaria through the use of the new synthetic insecticides? If so, which insecticides should be used; in what dosages and treatment cycles; at what financial costs; and in which zones? There was agreement that interventions were justified in zones of endemic malaria that were subject to epidemic outbreaks. The logic — and the potential consequences — of intervention with synthetic insecticides in regions of intense transmission, however, was in hot dispute.

Important malaria control experiences in African urban zones were accumulating. Malariologists had scored moderate successes in using synthetic larvicides, particularly to eliminate mosquito-breeding areas within African cities and towns and to maintain protective belts around urban agglomerations. House-spraying experiments with DDT had impressively reduced malarial infections, as had house spraying with benzene hexachloride (BHC).[26] Indeed, these experiences indicated that the way forward toward better control of malaria in rural Africa was likely going to be along the path of IRS. This meant a change in strategy: malaria control should target adult mosquitoes, rather than larvae.[27] A house-spraying project in southwestern Nigeria, using BHC, was already in progress. Its aim was to investigate the practicality of using IRS alone to create a malaria-free "island" in rural tropical Africa, in an extension of the practice of creating protective belts around urban agglomerations. The island was the town of Ilaro with 12,000 inhabitants, surrounded by secondary forest.[28]

The logic of an IRS intervention in rural Africa rested upon the assumptions that malaria imposed high economic costs, that the lifting of this burden would be necessary for economic growth and development, and that IRS would be the least expensive — indeed, the only practical — method of control.[29] Empirical

---

[25] Report of the Malaria Conference in Equatorial Africa, WHO/Mal/69, 41.

[26] Dr. F.J.C. Cambournac, Report on Malaria in Equatorial Africa, WHO/Mal/58, 21–6.

[27] Dr. F.J.C. Cambournac, Report on Malaria in Equatorial Africa, WHO/Mal/58, 32.

[28] The project had been suggested by the WHO Expert Committee on Malaria in 1948. See L.J. Bruce-Chwatt, The Ilaro Experimental Vector Species Eradication Scheme by Residual Insecticide Sparying (First Progress Report), 5 May 1950, WHO/MAL/40; L.J. Bruce-Chwatt, H. Archibald, R. Elliott, R.A. Fitz-John, and I.A. Balogus, Ilaro experimental malaria control scheme: report on four years' results, *Fifth International Congress on Tropical Medicine and Malaria*, 1953, **2** *Communications*, 54–66: Istanbul, 1953.

[29] For a general statement of the issues, see G. Macdonald, The Economic Importance of Malaria in Africa, 24 October 1950, WHO/MAL/60.

investigations were still in their early stages, but this logic was bolstered by the experiences with malaria control in the Transvaal, where the South African authorities reported an improvement in overall 'native' health and the loss of fewer workdays to sickness. The implication was that malaria control could be a profound stimulus to economic growth.

The second strand of reasoning was that the burden of malaria, as measured in childhood mortality, was unacceptably high. The actual extent of the childhood burden was unknown at the time, and professional opinion ranged widely.[30] Studies had begun in Nigeria, and the preliminary evidence suggested that malaria mightfully account for fully twenty-five percent of childhood deaths.[31] The extent of childhood medical problems caused or exacerbated by malaria was also unknown.

The experts all agreed, given the state of knowledge at the time, on the impossibility of recommending any standard protocol for malaria control for rural tropical Africa. As the final report stated, "The diversity of features of this continent is such that each project should be specially designed to meet the particular situation and to deal with it by the most satisfactory and economical way."[32]

Health gains from malaria interventions were evident in areas where the malaria burden was seasonal, the degree of acquired immunity was not robust, the average adult received relatively few inoculations per season, and the inoculations produced sickness. In this paper, Macdonald also attacked the views of malariologists who held that adult populations in 'hyperendemic' African regions had achieved a perfect balance with the malarial parasites.

[30]P.C.C. Garnham, one of the eminent British malariologists in East Africa, conducted post-mortem examinations on children in Kisumu, an area of hyperendemic transmission in Kenya. He concluded, in correspondence with his colleague Mr. Paterson, that malaria was rare as a cause of death: "These researches demonstrated the almost complete tolerance rapidly obtained against the parasite in practically all areas and the comparative rarity of Malaria as a cause of death. I have mentioned these observations because, from discussions with many Medical Officers, most appear to hold contrary views on the subject." [Prof. P.C.C. Garnham to Mr. Paterson, 1 June 1942, Native Hospital Kisumu. Correspondence. A.2. No. 11. Papers of Professor Percy Cyril Claude Garnham (1901–1995). Contemporary Medical Archives Centre, Wellcome Institute for the History of Medicine, London.] This position was one that Garnham had held for many years. In the 1930s, Garnham had argued for significant differences in placental malaria between West African and East African populations in regions of hyperendemicity. P.C.C. Garnham, Malaria in East Africa, a letter to the editor, *Transactions of the Royal Society of Tropical Medicine and Hygiene*, 24 March 1939.

Prof. George Macdonald, the Director of the Ross Institute at the London School of Hygiene and Tropical Medicine, was unimpressed with Garnham's interpretation of the Kisumu data and pointed out flaws in his work. George Macdonald to P.C.C. Garnham, 5 June 1950. PP/PCG/C22. Contemporary Medical Archives Centre, Wellcome Institute for the History of Medicine, London.

[31]Dr. F.J.C. Cambournac, Report on Malaria in Equatorial Africa, WHO/Mal/58, 44.

[32]Report of the Malaria Conference in Equatorial Africa, WHO/Mal/69, 46.

The WHO Project Sites

The experts expected that new technical challenges would arise in different African ecological settings. In preparation for the Kampala conference, Cambournac had compiled a list of the institutions concerned with malaria interventions and research, and this provided a rough overview of the interventions in progress. Post-Kampala conference, the role of the WHO malaria experts was to act as technical advisors on projects that would be supported with UNICEF funds, to investigate the possibility of moving from malaria control to the cessation of malaria transmission. The hope was that these pilot malaria eradication projects would be able to determine the most cost-effective application of the new synthetic insecticides and that these insecticides would fully interrupt malaria transmission. If the best and least expensive practices could be determined, it might be possible to 'scale-up' the pilot projects. If so, African colonies and states might undertake full-scale eradication programs similar to those unfolding on other continents burdened with malaria. The WHO pilot projects were launched in forest, savanna, sahelian, coastal, and highland zones in tropical Africa. Even before the Second World War, successful malaria control efforts had proved their worth on European-owned farms and plantations, around some of the mining centers, and in urban areas. In the early postwar years, several large-scale urban malaria control projects had experimented with IRS and larviciding using synthetic insecticides, and some produced promising results.[33] On the highland plateau of Madagascar, beginning in 1949, the French had launched an ambitious program of IRS and larviciding, combined with weekly chloroquine chemoprophylaxis for children under the age of 15. The results were dramatically reduced infections, suggesting the possibility of full, if local, eradication of malaria.[34]

One of the WHO pilot projects radiated out from Yaoundé in southern Cameroun in an effort to create a larger malaria-free zone that extended into the urban hinterland. The focus of the other pilot projects, however, was in rural zones. The long experience with urban and enclave malaria interventions suggested, at a minimum, that malaria infections could be dramatically reduced in these settings, given a sufficiently large outlay of funds. In rural areas — beyond

---

[33] As examples of a broad set of experiences, see G.A. Walton, On the control of malaria in Freetown, Sierra Leone. II. control methods and the effects upon the transmission of *Plasmodium Falciparum* resulting from the reduced abundance of *Anopheles Gambiae*, *Annals of Tropical Medicine and Parasitology*, 1949, **43**(2), 117–39; F. Merle and L. Maillot, Campagnes de désinsectisation contre le paludisme à Brazzaville, *Bulletin de la Société de Pathologie exotique et de ses filiales*, 1955, **48**(2), 242–69.

[34] G. Joncour, Present Situation in Regard to Malaria Control in Madagascar, 14 November 1955, WHO/MAL/150.

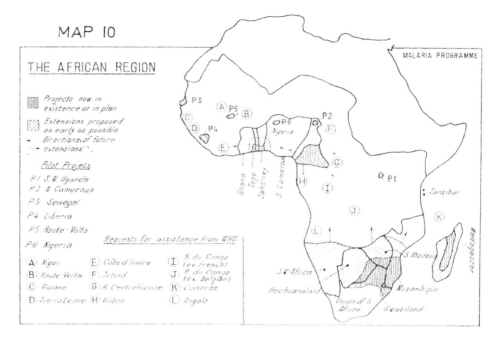

Figure 1. WHO malaria eradication pilot projects in 1960.

Source: AFRO MALARIA YEAR BOOK No. 2, Regional Office for Africa, WHO [1960].

the European farms and plantations — the charge was different. Where there was no prospect of securing funding for ongoing rural projects, and the focus of the projects was on a permanent solution. Would it be possible to fully interrupt the transmission of malaria at an affordable cost?

The malariologists' hopes for the complete interruption of malaria transmission sailed forward on the winds of optimism about the powers of the new synthetic insecticides. Whereas the success of the antimosquito measures of the earlier twentieth century had rested principally upon killing mosquito larva *in situ* and/or destroying mosquito habitat, the new generation of synthetic insecticides trumped the older generation on two counts. First, they were far less expensive. This meant that a given budget could be used to reach many more people. And second, at least some of the new insecticides, when sprayed on buildings, left behind long-acting residues. This raised hopes that per unit spraying costs would be dramatically lower.

In practice, the application of synthetic insecticides in tropical Africa was far from straightforward. The insecticides interacted with the house materials in unpredictable ways. Some modes of house construction required a great deal more insecticide than others, and on some house materials, emulsion sprays worked better than wettable powders. Rainy seasons wreaked havoc on the indoor residual sprays, and thus the cycle of sprayings — once, twice, thrice, or even twelve times a year — had to be worked out on an empirical basis.

The Entomological Labyrinth

The effective application of insecticides also depended upon an understanding of the behavior of the African mosquito vectors. At the time, little was known, and the experts at the 1950 Kampala conference agreed that basic research on the principal African vectors was essential. Their emphasis on the need for local entomological investigation as a basic foundation of malaria control was very much in line with the development of malariology elsewhere. It was part of what today would be called 'best practice.' In tropical Africa, local entomological studies proved greatly complex.

One key issue was the ecological range of the *Anopheles gambiae* mosquito. There was a long road ahead toward a fuller appreciation of the complexity of related species, with different behaviors and genetic susceptibilities to insecticides. Yet as researchers on the *Anopheles gambiae* complex made important advances and drew important distinctions, the role of entomology in the antimalaria projects was downgraded. As the killing powers of the synthetic insecticides in tropical Africa were brought to bear, mosquito research itself seemed less important: If the insecticides worked against all vector mosquitoes, what was the point of spending resources on understanding micro-variations in feeding, breeding, alighting, or other bionomic matters? A gulf began to open up between the entomologists and the project managers whose understanding of mosquito species was rudimentary at best.

Some basic mosquito behaviors appeared to be well enough understood to permit the pilot projects to move forward. A widely shared belief was that both *Anopheles gambiae* and *Anopheles funestus* were largely endophilic, that the female took her blood meal indoors. This was the foundational rationale for indoor residual spraying: When the female mosquito alights on a sprayed surface, either before or after she takes her blood meal, she would pick up enough insecticide to cause her death. Confidence in the indoor-resting, or endophilic, behavior of *Anopheles gambiae* and *Anopheles funestus* was strong. The behaviors of the other African anopheline vectors were less certain but seemed of only minor importance. It did not initially occur to the researchers that the two principal African vectors might have a range of specialized feeding and resting behaviors that could be influenced by IRS.

The Mixed Record of Synthetic Insecticides

In line with the recommendations of the Kampala conference and those of the Colonial Insecticides Committee in the U.K., the malaria control project managers experimented with a number of different synthetic pesticides. DDT and lindane (gamma-hexachlorocyclohexane, also known as gammexane or HCH)[35] had been used to

---

[35] In the malariological literature of the era, BHC was sometimes also referred to as gammexane.

control malaria in urban settings in a very minor role during the final years of the war and in a larger role beginning in 1945, at the transition from the use of the older generation of larvicides such as Paris Green (a copper arsunate) and 'malariol' (an oil).

The initial postwar experience with DDT in tropical Africa was mixed. In Monrovia, Liberia, for example, beginning in 1945, the Americans oversaw the spraying of DDT for both IRS and larvicidal purposes throughout the city and its surroundings. DDT spraying had little direct killing or residual effect because the house materials were sorptive. Houses had to be sprayed frequently, and the costs were prohibitive.[36] In Freetown, Sierra Leone, DDT, too, produced disappointing results.[37] The overall judgment of the Colonial Insecticides Committee in 1947 was negative: "…it appears that in its present form at least D.D.T. in Kerosene applied as a residual insecticide in West African village houses may not be of very great value in reducing the numbers and infectivity of *Anopheles*."[38] Greater success seemed to be promised by a shift to a new chlorinated hydrocarbon, first produced in 1948, known as dieldrin (DLD).

This was a common pattern throughout the West African projects: an experimental turn toward dieldrin, which had a long residual action like DDT, and, in some cases, toward benzene hexachloride (BHC). (HCH had a very weak residual action.) Both DLD and BHC produced a greater immediate 'kill rate' than did DDT. Yet mosquito resistance to DLD (which conveyed a cross-resistance to HCH) developed rapidly — often within a year or so of extensive use. Resistance was first noted in northwestern Nigeria in 1956 and by the early 1960s resistance had spread over a vast area of West Africa, from the Gambia and Mali to Congo and Northern Cameroon.[39] In 1961, cross-resistance between BHC and DLD

---

[36] Webb, First large-scale use, *op.cit.*

[37] As F. Maclagan, Acting Director of Medical Services, Medical Department, Freetown, put it: "The treatment of Freetown with D.D.T. solution has not prevented mosquito nuisance, and has had no measurable effect on room density indices. As a malaria control measure no form or residual insecticide has so far been shown to be effective under West African conditions." F. Maclagan, Use of D.D.T. as a Residual Insecticide for the Control of Malaria in Freetown, CO 554/153/1, National Archives of the U.K.

[38] Colonial Pesticides Committee, Summary of Experiments on the Effects of House Spraying with Pyrethrum and with D.D.T. in Kerosene on *A. Gambiae* and *A. Melas* in West Africa. Colonial Medical Research Committee, CIC (47) 3 C.M.R. (46) 72, 20th December 1946, CO 911/1, National Archives of the U.K.

[39] At Bernin Kebbi in northern Nigeria, the Shell Oil Company, which produced dieldrin, continued to promote its use, even after major problems emerged. As Dr. James Haworth, the chief administrator of the malaria control project in Bernin Kebbi, wrote of his experiences there, "…it brought me in touch with the worst form of commercialism as practised by Shell who sold one of the insecticides used. In spite of all scientific evidence, they refused to accept the fact that dieldrin was an extremely persistent poison affecting both animals and humans and that it quickly lost its effectiveness as the *Anopheline* mosquitoes (and most other insects) rapidly acquired a resistance to the chemical."

emerged in northern Cameroon, and for the first time in tropical Africa, also in northern Cameroon, researchers documented vector resistance to DDT.[40] In the following years, experts suspected that DDT resistance had also emerged in Senegal and in Congo, although this seemed to be of little practical significance; in many West African projects, the use of DDT had not been able to interrupt the transmission of malaria.[41]

These West African experiences with synthetic insecticides differed from those in East Africa. There, *Anopheles gambiae* and the other malaria vectors did not develop resistance to either DLD or BHC. The absence of this constraint meant that there was less need for experimentation. The pilot project at Kigezi in Uganda used DDT exclusively; the malaria control project at Pare-Taveta on the Kenya/Tanzanian border never used DDT.[42] These West and East African experiences differed, in turn, from those in southern Africa. There, the vectors were less efficient; the house materials were less problematic for spraying on insecticides; malaria transmission was markedly seasonal; and the levels of endemicity were low. The malaria control services based their successful programs upon the indoor spraying of houses with BHC as well as DDT.[43]

The Loss of Acquired Immunities and Epidemic 'Rebound' Malaria

At the Kampala conference, the unresolved question of the health consequences of the loss of acquired immunities in populations living in areas of heavy endemic

---

[Dr. James Haworth, Development Records Project — Nigeria; Dr. James Haworth 1947–1958, 9, MSS. Afr. s. 1872 (73), Rhodes House, Oxford, U.K.

[40] Ph. Cavalié and J. Mouchet, The Experimental Malaria Eradication Campaign in the North of the Republic of Cameroon. II. Antimalaria Operations and Their Results, 8 December 1961, WHO/MAL/323, 21.

[41] J. Mouchet and J. Hamon, Les problèmes techniques de l'éradication du paludisme en Afrique, *Médecine tropicale et paludisme*, 1963, 39–48; J. Coz and J. Hamon, Importance pratique de la résistance aux insecticides en Afrique au sud du Sahara pour l'éradication du paludisme dans ce continent, *Cahiers O.R.S.T.O.M.*, Entomologie Médicale, 1963, (1), 27–37; J. Hamon and J. Mouchet, La résistance aux insecticides chez les insects d'importance médicale. Méthodes d'étude et situation en Afrique au sud du Sahara, *Médecine tropicale*, 1961, 21(5), 565–96.

[42] J. Mouchet and J. Hamon, Difficulties in Malaria Eradication Campaigns Due to the Behaviour of the Vectors, 16 May 1963, WHO/MAL/394, 7; J. Hamon, Insecticide-Resistance in Major Vectors of Malaria, and Its Operational Significance, 22 March 1962, WHO/MAL/336, 12.

[43] [n.a.], Malaria in the African Region. A Review, 20 August 1958, WHO AFRO/MAL/2, 9. Later, DDT resistance in the Transvaal and DDT, DLD, and HCH resistance in Swaziland emerged. See the WHO map, Countries with Insecticide Resistance in *Anopheles* Mosquitoes of Particular Importance, held by the WHO archives in Geneva. [Undated, it has no formal finding code and is filed with WHO disease maps.]

transmission as a result of malaria interventions had been explosive.[44] Childhood morbidity and mortality were conceptualized as "costs" that were paid to acquire adult and adolescent immunity. How high were the "costs" of the acquisition of immunity? What was the extent of childhood morbidity and mortality that was attributable to malaria? The advocates for greater caution buttressed their arguments with the assumptions that childhood mortality costs in areas of heavy endemic transmission were relatively low. The implication — contested by their opponents — was that these putatively low childhood mortality costs might be an acceptable price for fully functional adult immunity.

In the aftermath of Kampala, in the early 1950s the medical community moved closer to a consensus on the high costs of childhood mortality. An estimate of 25 percent of childhood mortality directly attributable to malaria came to be more widely accepted, and thus, for those who accepted this estimate, one of the reasons for caution in malaria intervention dissipated. By virtue of the good that could be conveyed to those in the early years of life through the prevention of malaria transmission, the concern over the harm that might be done to adults, in areas of heavy transmission whose acquired immunities had been compromised through malaria interventions, went to the back burner.

This issue of acquired immunities to *falciparum* malaria had salience principally in tropical Africa. It was not a major issue in the broader global campaign to eradicate malaria (1955–1969) because on no other subcontinent region was principally *falciparum* transmission maintained at such high levels. For this reason, the ethics of partially successful malaria intervention went unexplored: the unstated assumption was that malaria intervention was an obvious and unequivocal good because it saved lives and prevented illness. With enthusiasm for the prospects for full success, malariologists were not drawn to an exploration of the consequences of only partial success or of the lapsing of control measures. This was a significant oversight, because in some instances in tropical Africa when malaria control or eradication projects in areas of heavy endemic transmission lapsed — which was nearly invariably the case — those whose acquired immunities had been compromised bore a

---

[44]At the Kampala conference, new definitions were agreed to distinguish between levels of heavy endemic transmission in which there were different percentages of the population with distended spleens. The areas in which the spleen rate in children of 2–10 years of age was constantly over 50 percent and in which the spleen rate in adults was "high" were to be classified as *hyperendemic*; those areas in which the spleen rate in children of 2–10 years of age was constantly over 75 percent and in which the spleen rate in adults was "low" were to be classified as *holoendemic*. The "strongest adult tolerance" to malaria was said to be found in holoendemic regions. Report on the Malaria Conference in Equatorial Africa, World Health Organization Technical Report Series, no. 38, World Health Organization, 1951, 45: Geneva. Malariologists later discovered regions of heavy endemic malaria transmission in which the spleen rates of the populations did not accord well with these definitional criteria.

suddenly increased burden of death and disease. The 'rebound' malaria epidemics that followed on the heels of the malaria interventions in Africa produced an increase in human suffering in a different age cohort from those who benefited from the interventions. It was noble to save the life of a child. What was the moral accounting when the rebound epidemic malaria from a lapsed intervention struck down the father, mother, or grandparent?

Little was known about the natural course of malaria infections in tropical Africa. How long did it take for acquired immunities to degrade? Did they degrade fully or only partially?[45] Some clinical studies advanced evidence showed that individuals reinfected after having been resident in an antimalaria pilot project zone might be free of malaria symptoms; yet the fact of asymptomatism suggested to others that the interventions had not continued long enough to cause a fuller degradation of immune status. In the aftermath of the pilot project near Yaoundé, epidemic malaria produced symptoms of acute malaria that had only exceptionally been previously recorded.[46] In the aftermath of the pilot project in the Kpain region of central Liberia, epidemic malaria surged through the once protected communities.[47] When 'rebound' epidemic malaria struck, the disease consequences went unmeasured. Although the Kampala conference had recommended that malaria control services be established to allow for effective intervention in the case of rebound malaria, this recommendation had not been implemented. The malaria control projects had not been charged to create a malaria service or any other type of public health infrastructure, and the institutional capacities for medical surveillance in tropical Africa in the 1950s were rudimentary at best.

Antimalarial Drugs and the Pilot Projects

By the mid 1950s, as the evidence began to accumulate from the first cluster of pilot projects that IRS alone would not be able to interrupt transmission, malariologists

---

[45]L.J. Bruce-Chwatt investigated the state of knowledge of this issue in his 1962 report, A Longitudinal Survey of Natural Malaria Infection in a Group of West African Adults, 17 December 1962, WHO/MAL/369. This work was also published as, A longitudinal survey of natural malaria infection in a group of West African adults. I, *West African Medical Journal,* 1963, **12**, 141–73; and, A longitudinal survey of natural malaria infection in a group of West African adults. II, *West African Medical Journal,* 1963, **12**, 199–217.

Bruce-Chwatt was a well-known advocate for the expansion of indoor residual spraying in tropical Africa, and at the Kampala conference he had championed the interventionist position. In his 1962 report, he found that the evidence about the medical consequences of lapsed intervention was mixed and difficult to interpret.

[46]Bruce-Chwatt, A Longitudinal Survey, *op.cit.* WHO/MAL/369, 62.

[47]Webb, First large-scale use, *op.cit.*

designed the second cluster of projects either with a chemoprophylactic or chemo-therapeutic component or both.[48] At a WHO technical meeting on African malaria held in Brazzaville in 1957, the malaria experts unanimously recommended the initiation of large-scale experiments with the mass administration of antimalarials. The recommendation was to employ different drugs and dosage schedules, in order to determine the efficacy of the interventions.[49]

The mass administration of antimalarial drugs had a long and checkered history into the mid-twentieth century. The Italians had undertaken the first national mass drug administration program, with mixed success. In a mixed malarial environment of *vivax*, *falciparum*, and *malariae* infections, the mass administration of quinine had dramatically reduced malarial deaths, but not morbidity.[50]

In tropical Africa before the Second World War, there had been no comparable experience with mass drug administration of quinine. The British and French colonial powers had set up cinchona plantations during the interwar years, but the quantities of cinchona alkaloids produced had been small. Some Africans, particularly those living in urban areas, acquired quinine through post office sales of individual doses, but the number of individuals who availed themselves of this chemical therapy was relatively small. From a public health point of view, the scant local supplies and the high cost of quinine on the international market had excluded the option of mass campaigns. There was, furthermore, an underlying disquiet about the use of quinine to protect tropical Africans: some malariologists believed that quinine could disturb the mechanism of immunity and subsequently produce more severe malarial problems.[51] P.C.C. Garnham, for example, held that the provision of quinine prophylaxis for populations in areas of heavy endemic transmission who had been exposed to various strains of malaria was unnecessary and its prolonged use could do harm.[52]

---

[48] Max J. Miller, Chemotherapy in Malaria Control, 20 September 1955, WHO/MAL/137; I.H. Vincke, Place of Chemotherapy in Modern Malaria Control Programs, 27 October 1955, WHO/MAL/147; L.J. Bruce-Chwatt, Chemotherapy in Relation to Possibilities of Malaria Eradication in Tropical Africa, 21 May 1956, WHO/MAL/175.

[49] M.A.C. Dowling, The Use of Mass Drug Administration in Malaria Projects in the African Region, [n.d.; circa 1961], AFR/MAL/39, 1.

[50] Snowden, *The Conquest of Malaria, op.cit.*, 53–114.

[51] M. Robert, M. le Médecin Général Inspecteur, Directeur Général de la Santé Publique en A.O.F. à M. le Directeur des Affaires Economiques et du Plan (Bureau de la Production des Exportations et des Prix), [n.d. (1955), reçu 14 novembre 1955], 1-3, Dossier Antipaludiques, Box 232, Archives de l'Institut de Médecine Tropicale du Service de Santé des Armées (IMTSSA), Marseilles; Le Médecin Général Inspecteur, Directeur de la Santé Publique en A.O.F., Note au sujet de: La Quinine dans la lutte antipalustre en A.O.F., [n.d., circa 1955], 3, Dossier Antipaludiques, Box 232, Archives de l'Institut de Médecine Tropicale du Service de Santé des Armées (IMTSSA), Marseilles.

[52] P.C.C. Garnham, Quinine Prophylaxis for European and African troops, 12 December 1939. PP/PCG/C5, Papers of Professor Percy Cyril Claude Garnham (1901–1995), Contemporary Medical Archives Centre, Wellcome Institute for the History of Medicine, London.

In the postwar period, the availability of synthetic drugs opened up a new world of possibilities for malaria interventions. The synthetic drugs pyrimethamine and chloroquine seemed to have fewer side effects than quinine.[53] Both could serve either as a malaria prophylaxis or a cure. As the price of the synthetic drugs dropped, their sheer inexpensiveness allowed malariologists to consider deploying the drugs in new roles. They might limit the damage from outbreaks of epidemic malaria in highland areas in which African populations had little or no immunity; interrupt transmission before or during an IRS campaign; protect the young in the absence of other efforts to control malaria; and/or reduce malaria during the transmission season, whether or not other control efforts were on-going. If the insecticides alone were capable of greatly reducing but not completely interrupting transmission, the drugs might be able to clean up the 'human reservoir' of parasites and perhaps reach the goal of zero transmission. Another vision was that of regular, ongoing mass chemoprophylaxis.[54]

---

[53]As M. Robert, M. le Médecin Général Inspecteur, Directeur Général de la Santé Publique en A.O.F., put it: "Certains essais de chimio-prophylaxie de mass par la quinine et même dans certains cas par les synthétiques, ont fait apparaître la fièvre bilieuse hémoglobinurique avec une grande fréquence chez les africains, alors que cetter affection était extrêmement rare chex eux avant l'introduction des anti-malariques et était réservée à l'européen non immunisé par les infections de l'enfance et soumis a une prophylaxie quinuinique mal appliquée ."

"Il est remarkable, et ceci est démontré par les statistiques, comme par l'expérience des médecins des hôpitaux d'A.O.F., que la fièvre bilieuse hémoglobinurique est en voie de disparition depuis l'utilisation de la chimio-prophylaxie individuelle des produits synthéthiques.

"Appliquer à l'africain une chimio-prophylaxie quininque généralisée serait, dans les conditions actuelles, aboutir, non à l'éradication du paludisme — puisque les conditions de transmission persisteraient — mais à une dimunition dangereuse de son remarkable pouvoir de résistance vis-à-vis des complications sévères du paludisme." Institut de Médecine Tropicale du Service de Santé des Armées, Archives de l'Ecole du Pharo, Marseille, Box 232. Dossier Antipaludiques. M. Robert, M. le Médecin Général Inspecteur, Directeur Général de la Santé Publique en A.O.F., "Note au sujet de: La Quinine dans la lutte anti-palustre en A.O.F.," 3.

[54]The French had a different view of the prospects for mass antimalarial prophylaxis than did the British. In 1949, the French launched an extensive program of malaria control on the island of Madagascar that used mass chemoprophylaxis, and this interest was extended to their antimalaria projects on the mainland. The French medical legacy continued after independence: Cameroon and Senegal developed national antimalaria chemoprophylaxis programs. A.B.G. Laing, The impact of malaria chemoprophylaxis in Africa with special reference to Madagascar, Cameroon, and Senegal, *Bulletin of the World Health Organization,* 1984, **62**(Suppl), 41–8.

The British never developed such programs in their African colonies, and neither did any of the independent African states that gained their independence from the British. British view was that regular prophylaxis did not make much sense in tropical Africa because the high rate of malaria transmission (in conjunction with a concern about compromising the immunological status of Africans) meant that a regime of prophylaxis would demand high levels of compliance, and this was deemed unachievable.

A major challenge was in getting drugs to the rural populations within a project zone. One option was mixing antimalarial medicines into sodium chloride, on the theory that everybody consumed salt. Moderately large-scale distributions of chloroquine-medicated salt were introduced into a zone of 30,000 people in northern Ghana and into communities of laborers with a total population of over 23,000 who worked on two sugar estates in Uganda. Both programs ran into insurmountable difficulties, including the rejection (or non-use) of the medicated salt.[55] A trial in Tanzania, in a region in which the supply of salt could be completely controlled, in conjunction with a successful health propaganda campaign, produced a short-term medical success.[56]

In Bobo-Dioulasso in Upper Volta and at Bernin Kebbi in northern Nigeria, project managers oversaw the direct distribution of antimalarial tablets to the Africans in the project zones. An alternate approach was via unmonitored direct distribution — which meant providing drugs to village heads or other local authorities that in turn distributed them. In Uganda and in northern Cameroon, the project authorities tried a monitored distribution of a single-dose of antimalarial drug during the spraying cycle, and this approach succeeded in further reducing the parasite prevalence. Monitored distribution, however, proved too costly to be 'scaled-up.' In Madagascar, Ghana, and Senegal, there were programs of unmonitored direct distribution of antimalarials for long-term prophylaxis. Costs were lower, but the effectiveness of distribution diminished quickly, and the programs ran the risks of inadvertent overdosing.

Researchers judged the overall results of the chemotherapeutic interventions to be unimpressive. In monitored distribution schemes in Upper Volta, northern Cameroon, Ghana, and northern Nigeria, pyrimethamine was initially highly efficacious, but it produced resistance in the *falciparum* parasite within a few months. Chloroquine alone or in combination with primaquine also cleared infections, but the prospects for long-term prophylaxis were poor. The major impediment — nearly insuperable — was the establishment of a regular rhythm of distribution and use. Moreover, the utility of mass drug distribution schemes was called into question by their apparent inability to achieve project goals. In combination with IRS, antimalarial drugs could drive rates of infection extremely low, but not to the point of fully interrupting transmission.[57]

---

[55] S.A. Hall and N.E. Wilks, A trial of chloroquine-medicated salt for malaria suppression in Uganda, *American Journal of Tropical Medicine and Hygiene*, 1967, **16**(4), 429–42; [n.a.], Assessment Report on the Ghana-18 Medicated Salt Pilot Project, 2, SJ 5, JKT 1, Ghana, WHO7.0017, WHO Archives, Geneva.

[56] D.F. Clyde, Suppression of malaria in Tanzania with the use of medicated salt, *Bulletin of the World Health Organization*, 1966, **35**(6), 962–8.

[57] J. Hamon, J. Mouchet, and G. Chauvet. Bilan de quatorze années de lutte contre le paludisme dans les pays francophones d'Afrique tropicale et à Madagascar. Considérations sur la persistance de la

The Lessons of the Malaria Control and Eradication Projects

In the early 1960s, after years of effort that had protected millions of Africans, the WHO malariologists closed down the pilot projects. They had accumulated a wealth of practical experience across tropical Africa. They had analyzed data on morbidity and mortality, mosquitoes, parasites, spleen-rates, fevers, and insecticides, and they had grappled with the organizational challenges of indoor residual housespraying and the distribution of antimalarial drugs. The malariologists had sought to develop eradication protocols that, subject to local conditions, could be used across the continent.

The malariologists had been little attuned to the African social universes in whose midst their antimalaria projects unfolded, and the projects advanced largely without input from the communities in the project zones. The cultural gulf remained fundamentally unbridged. The project workers discovered that many Africans were not interested in ingesting salt laced with antimalarials and that many were unwilling to take regular doses of prophylactic pills. Many Africans became fatigued with the household disruptions that accompanied the cycles of IRS, and after the sprayed insecticides stopped working against household bugs and vermin, some closed their doors to the spray teams.

The malariologists were also unprepared for the extent of the movement of people between a project zone and its surrounding region. The project zones had been established as territorial blocs, with 'treated' areas adjoining 'untreated' zones that served to provide baseline data. The population movements confounded the malariologists' work, because parasitized individuals from unsprayed areas reignited malarial infections in villages where transmission had been reduced to near zero. The problem became complicated further when people moved across state boundaries.

The issue of migration had daunting proportions: it meant that malarial infections could be introduced and exchanged across virtually the entirety of sub-Saharan Africa. (Sub-Saharan *falciparum* infections were unable to gain a footing in Europe, owing to the lack of susceptibility of the Mediterranean vectors to the African genotypes.) Any antimalaria campaign that aimed at zero transmission would require the cooperation of the governments in the adjoining states. This was a tremendous challenge, because the newly independent governments (and the central governments of Liberia and Ethiopia) had little effective reach into large parts of their state territories. And if national governments were weak, a successful antimalaria campaign would have to engage the energies and interests of the

transmission et perspectives d'avenir, *Bulletin de la Société de Pathologie exotique,* septembre-octobre 1963, **56**(5), 945–6.

indigenous political authorities. This was a large charge, because the cultural gaps in perception about the significance of malaria were great.

The eradication campaign had been driven by the insights and assumptions of Western bioscience. The Western perceptions of the seriousness of malaria were honed by knowledge of the vulnerability of non-immunes in tropical Africa, economic arguments about the loss of worker productivity, and growing evidence that malaria killed many African children and wreaked havoc with the lives of some who survived. African perceptions were very different. Africans thought about the serious complications of malaria for children using very different cosmological frameworks from those of the Western-trained biomedical workers.[58] Moreover, most Africans thought of the childhood afflictions as quite distinct from the fevers and flu-like symptoms experienced by Africans who had achieved robust levels of acquired immunity. For African adults, malaria was largely perceived as an annoyance, an unpleasant reality of life like the seasonal flu, rather than a vital problem to be tackled with scarce resources. At independence, most African states declined to take up the "pre-eradication" programs recommended by the World Health Organization.

On the technical side, the antimalaria projects demonstrated that indoor spraying with residual insecticides and the use of antimalarial drugs to prevent or to clear infections at the population level could greatly reduce the transmission of malaria but could not reduce the levels to zero. One lesson drawn from the projects was thus that the malaria eradication in tropical Africa was not feasible, given the extant tools, resources, and constraints. The corollary was that malaria control was feasible and that it might be achieved if Africans prioritized malaria as a critically important health issue. The issue of the financial sustainability of long-term malaria control remained moot because, except in a few areas of southern Africa, long-term programs were not put in place.

The control and eradication projects also pointed toward the conclusion that residual insecticides could not be used indefinitely to control malaria. All of the insecticides — HHC, BHC, DLD, and to a lesser extent DDT — had been selected for mosquito resistance. The antimalarial drugs appeared to operate similarly in a parallel domain. The mass use of the drug pyrimethamine had quickly selected for parasite resistance, and it seemed that other antimalarials might eventually do the same. Although in 1965 widespread *falciparum* resistance to chloroquine in tropical Africa lay some years in the future, some prescient malariologists anticipated its emergence.

---

[58] See, for example, Alma Gottlieb, *The Afterlife Is Where We Come From: The Culture of Infancy in West Africa*, University of Chicago Press, 2004: Chicago.

4 The Use and Misuse of History: Lessons from Sardinia

Frank M. Snowden

Introduction

In 1944–45, as the Second World War ended and the Cold War began, Italy experienced a massive epidemic of malaria driven by the devastating social, economic, and environmental consequences of warfare. This epidemic struck Sardinia, the most malarious Italian region, with special severity. In a population of 794,000 some 78,173 fell ill in 1944, suffering primarily from malignant tertian malaria caused by *Plasmodium falciparum,* which peaked in the summer and autumn. Fevers due to *Plasmodium vivax* predominated in the spring, and mixed infections of both were common.[1] This public health emergency furnished an occasion for the scientists of the Rockefeller Foundation — "a long-awaited opportunity to begin serious health work in Europe," as they described it.[2] The International Health Division of the Foundation had long been involved in the global effort to control malaria, and as early as 1925 it had adopted Italy as a base for its research. Its members welcomed the opportunity to undertake the experiment of eradicating the disease from Sardinia while also providing an arresting display of the power of American technology. Rockefeller scientists persuaded the American and Italian governments to implement their war-inspired strategy. The idea was to

---

[1] A survey of the postwar epidemic is Paul F. Russell, Memorandum on Malaria and Its Control in Liberated Italy, 1 January - 30 September 1944, 11 October 1944. Rockefeller Archive Center (RAC), Record Group 1.2, Series 700 Europe, box 12, folder 101, Rockefeller Foundation Health Commission, 1944 (February - October).

[2] W.A. Sawyer, Inter-office memo to R.B.F., April 17, 1944. RAC, Record Group 1.2, Series 700 Europe, box 12, folder 101, Rockefeller Foundation Health Commission, 1944 (February - October).

follow the victorious war against the Axis powers with a new military campaign to annihilate a species of insect.

The target was the mosquito *Anopheles labranchiae,* the much feared vector principally responsible for transmitting malaria in the region. The Rockefeller malariologist Fred Soper had succeeded in eradicating the invasive species of mosquito *Anopheles gambiae* in Brazil and Egypt in order to halt the transmission of yellow fever and malaria. Never before, however, had the attempt been made to exterminate an indigenous anopheline. This new experiment, known as the Sardinian Project, was planned in 1945 and launched in 1946 under the auspices of a specially created agency known as ERLAAS (Regional Entity for the Anti-Anopheline Battle in Sardinia). The effort continued until 1951, when it achieved a permanent victory over the ancient scourge. Sardinia was declared malaria-free in 1952 — for the first time, the Foundation reported, "since the arrival of the Phoenicians in 1200 B.C. [sic.]."[3] Small numbers of *Anopheles labranchiae* survived the onslaught, but the transmission of plasmodia was halted.

Ironically, the Sardinian Project triumphed not only over malaria but also over the indigenous traditions of Italian medical science and public health. For nearly the first half of the twentieth century the global field of malariology had been dominated by the so-called "Italian School" led by such figures as Angelo Celli, Giovanni Battista Grassi, and Ettore Marchiafava. Having unraveled many of the secrets of the etiology, epidemiology, and pathology of the disease, these scientists launched a national campaign to conquer malaria. Beginning at the turn of the century and lasting for decades, the Italian campaign relied on a patient, multifaceted program combining health education, chemotherapy, environmental sanitation, social uplift, and agricultural improvement.[4] The American intervention in Sardinia marked the rejection of this approach through reliance instead on a sudden assault with DDT as its single weapon of choice. This approach embodied what the Rockefeller expert W.L. Hackett in the 1930s termed the "American thesis" that malaria could be vanquished by employing technology alone to eradicate mosquitoes, thereby halting the transmission of malaria but obviating the need to address complex social and economic issues.[5] To apply this strategic vision, however, Hackett would have required a weapon far more powerful than

---

[3] RAC, Record Group 1.2, Series 700 Europe, box no. 12, folder 101 (Rockefeller Health Commission). Trustees' Confidential Bulletin, Fighting Malaria in Europe and Africa, 13.

[4] On the history of the Italian School and the campaign to eradicate malaria, see my work, *The Conquest of Malaria: Italy, 1900–1962,* Yale University Press, 2006: New Haven. An excellent account of the campaign in the regional context of Sardinia is Eugenia Tognotti, *Per una storia della malaria in Italia: Il caso della Sardegna,* 2nd ed., Franco Angeli, 2008: Milan.

[5] For Hackett's statement of the "American thesis", see, *Malaria in Europe: An Ecological Study,* Oxford University Press, 1937, 15–6: Oxford and London.

the arsenic-based preparation Paris Green, the most potent insecticide then available. With the discovery of a far more powerful residual poison and larvicide, it was tempting to suspect that the intricate mysteries of malaria could, as Hackett had indicated, be reduced to "an entomological rather than a social problem" that could now be resolved by means of DDT alone — the "atomic bomb of the insect world."[6]

Although DDT had been synthesized in 1874, its unrivalled insecticidal properties were discovered only in 1939 by the chemist Paul Müller, and tested in Italy. The first large-scale demonstration of its power took place in December 1943 and January 1944. It was used at that time to contain an epidemic of typhus at Naples by destroying the lice that transmit it when 3,000,000 people and their clothes were dusted with the hydrocarbon. After this success against lice, DDT was employed experimentally against mosquitoes at Castel Volturno, and subsequently in the Pontine Marshes and the Tiber Delta, where extensive flooding of the area by the retreating German army had led to a vast upsurge in malaria.[7] Success in these early trials prompted enthusiasm for the larger and more systematic deployment of the chemical in Sardinia, whose geographical isolation and moderate size approximating the area of the state of New Hampshire appealed to experimenters.

Victory in Sardinia marked the ascendance of the "American School" of malariology with its stress on technology over the once dominant "Italian School" whose approach had stressed the social, educational, and environmental determinants of disease. The triumphant narrative of this "American School" victory in Sardinia dominated the official history of the five-year spraying campaign. This work — The *Sardinian Project* — was written by its director, the sanitary engineer John Logan, in 1953.[8] Logan described in detail this pioneering attempt to destroy

---

[6] Hackett, *Malaria in Europe, op. cit.*,108; Margaret Humphreys, *Malaria: Poverty, Race, and Public Health in the United States*, 2001, 147: Baltimore.

[7] Fred Soper, The Use of DDT against Malaria Evaluated on a Risk-Benefit Basis, 3 December 1970. National Library of Medicine (NLM), Soper Papers, MS box 52. Cf. also Thomas H.G. Aitken, A Study of Winter DDT House-Spraying and Its Concomitant Effect on *Anophelines* and Malaria in an Endemic Area, 5 October 1945. NLM, Soper Papers, MS box 54.

[8] John A. Logan, *The Sardinian Project: An Experiment in the Eradication of an Indigenous Malaria Vector*, Johns Hopkins Press, 1953: Baltimore. Other histories of the Sardinian Project include P.J. Brown, Failure-as-sucess: multiple meanings of eradication in the Rockefeller Foundation Sardinian Project, 1946–1951, *Parassitologia*, 1998, 40(1–2), 117–30; J.A. Farley, Mosquitoes or malaira? Rockefeller campaigns in the American South and Sardinia, *Parassitologia*, 1994, 36(1–2), 165–73; Eugenia Tognotti, *Americani, comunisti e zanzare: Il piano di eradicazione della malaria in Sardegna tra scienza e politica negli anni della guerra fredda*, EDES, 1946–1950, 1995: Sassari; and, *La malaria in Sardegna: Per una storia del paludismo nel Mezzogiorno, 1880–1950*, F. Angeli,1996: Milan.

malaria by eradicating mosquitoes — an approach that, he predicted, would forever "push forward the frontiers of public health practice." Indeed, his prediction came true under the inspiration of the foremost Rockefeller malariologists — Fred Soper, the eradicator of mosquitoes in Brazil and in Egypt, and Paul Russell, the Chief Malariologist of the Allied Control Commission in Italy as the war ended. Echoing Logan's account of the power of DDT, Russell proclaimed *Man's Mastery of Malaria* and urged the Eighth World Health Assembly, meeting at Mexico City in 1955, to launch an unprecedently ambitious program.[9] Explicitly invoking the Sardinian experience in the discussion, Marcolino Gomes Candau, the Director-General of the World Health Organization (WHO), called on the Assembly to establish a global malaria eradication program using DDT as its weapon of choice and a one-size-fits-all methodology.[10] Directing the WHO effort that resulted, Emilio Pampana intended to reach the goal by exterminating mosquitoes according to a textbook strategy of four standardized steps — "preparation, attack, consolidation, and maintenance."[11]

The WHO campaign, unlike the Sardinian Project, ultimately foundered, and it was abandoned as a failure in 1969.[12] By then, however, malariology had ushered in a period of unparalleled hubris that dominated the entire field of infectious disease. Between 1945 and the recognition of the importance of emerging and re-emerging diseases in the 1990s, infectious diseases were thought to be easily eradicable as the industrial world crossed the threshold into an infection-free garden of Eden. Led first by malariology, the prevailing reasoning held that technology — and American technology in particular — could be counted on to develop weapons of such power as to eliminate communicable diseases one by one until they had all been eradicated.[13] The experiment in Sardinia thus helped to foster the expectation that the global conquest of all infections would be swift and painless with little need to address complex social and environmental problems.

Public health policy, therefore, needs to be informed by history. A policy that either ignores the lessons of the past or draws misguided lessons from it can all too easily result in serious mistakes and a colossal waste of resources. The WHO

---

[9] *Man's Mastery of Malaria*, 1955: New York.

[10] World Health Organization: Eighth World Health Assembly, Malaria Eradication: A Proposal by the Director-General, 3 May 1955, NLM, Soper Papers, MS box 55.

[11] *Textbook of Malaria Eradication*, 2nd ed., 1969: London.

[12] A brief history of the WHO campaign is M.A. Farid, The malaria program — from euphoria to anarchy, *World Health Forum* I, 1980, 8–22.

[13] Leading statements of the eradicationist belief are E.H. Hinman, *World Eradication of Infectious Diseases*, 1969: Springfield, IL; Aidan Cockburn, The *Evolution and Eradication of Infectious Diseases*, 1963: Johns Hopkins; and F. Burnett and D.O. White, *Natural History of Infectious Disease*, 4th ed., 1972: Cambridge.

demonstrated this danger when it embodied a misreading of Sardinian history in its global eradication program.

The purpose of this chapter is to re-examine the Sardinian Project and the boundless confidence in DDT that it inspired. The tendency to celebrate the Sardinian display of the power of DDT in isolation has long obscured a more complex and nuanced history. The result has been to nourish belief in magic bullets and in vector control as a stand-alone antimalarial methodology. The argument here is that success in Sardinia was based on a more complex set of initiatives than Logan, Soper, Russell, and the WHA have suggested. DDT was a useful and potent tool, but it was only one in a multifactorial approach that yielded victory.

Malaria and Sardinia as Synonyms

Malaria had afflicted Sardinia since antiquity, but — as for Italy as a whole — the late nineteenth century marked a vast upsurge in its ravages.[14] As the leading historian of malaria on the island writes, "The extraordinary tightness of the vice in which malaria held Sardinia by the end of the century was a recent phenomenon that emerged ... after national unification."[15] The very symbols of modernity and progress — national unification, railroads, and demographic growth — combined to create the environmental catastrophe of deforestation, which in turn had dire consequences for public health. With a rugged terrain dominated by hills and mountains punctuated by countless torrents and river valleys, and with an agriculture characterized by extensive small peasant farming, Sardinia had a hydrological system that was immensely vulnerable to the destruction of its woods and forests. Following the heavy rains of the late winter and spring, the rivers and torrents flooded their banks, only to dry up almost completely during the summer. In both flood and drought, they left stagnant pools both in their beds and in the adjacent countryside that they overran. Since the topsoil consisted of impermeable clay, pools of water did not drain away, but collected in innumerable depressions and hollows.

Population growth, the privatization of the land entailing the loss of common land and use rights, and the pressure of the onerous and regressive tax system of the new Liberal regime impelled peasants to clear ever higher slopes to plant wheat on virgin soil that was fertile for a period until it succumbed to erosion. At the same time the growth of railroads and a national market provided a vast market for lumber as well as the means to remove it. The result was a general invasion of

---

[14] The classic history of malaria in Sardinia is Eugenia Tognotti, *Per una storia della malaria in Italia: Il caso della Sardegna,* 2nd ed., Franco Angeli, 2008: Milan.
[15] *Ibid.,* 23.

the hills with axes, fire, mattocks, and plows. Herds of goat and sheep frequently completed the work of destruction with the final decimation of forests of beech, pine, chestnut, and oak that had once performed multiple functions in the regulation of the flow of water. The canopy broke the force of falling water and reduced its volume by providing broad leaf surfaces for evaporation. At the same time roots and undergrowth anchored the clay topsoil and protected the underlying limestone from the eroding forces of wind and rain. Drenched by spring downpours in the absence of this cover, the progressively denuded slopes generated torrents that swept away soil and rock, set off landslides, and silted up riverbeds downstream. Fed in this manner by rushes of water, soil, and detritus, rivers and streams repeatedly overflowed to unprecedented extents, creating stagnant ponds in valleys and along the coast. The report from the health council at Oristano commented on the process at work in the 1880s:

> Sardinia, which was once rich as a result of its ancient and flourishing forests, is now becoming a desert steppe through the vandalism of greedy speculators. Through love of lucre they are transforming into charcoal an immense number of plants that represent the patient legacy of centuries.

Since agriculture itself was backward and provided few countervailing opportunities to anchor the soil or control drainage, the result was the creation of countless expanses of stagnant or slow-moving water that were ideal for the breeding of mosquitoes. The scouts employed by the Sardinian Project recorded over a million such breeding places at all altitudes, but above all in the valleys and narrow coastal plains where the soil was most fertile and to which the population of peasants and farm laborers commuted at the height of the agricultural and malarial seasons. The degraded environment of the island was idea for the primary vector on the island — *Anopheles labranchiae*. This mosquito could breed in mountains pools up to altitudes of 3,000 feet, on the edges of streams and rivers, and in both fresh and brackish water along the coastline. By day it rested, and by night it feasted with a pronounced preference for human blood.

Anophelines also took advantage of opportunities that developed underground with the development of the mining industry that exploited deposits of lead, zinc, iron, silver, copper, antimony, and manganese in the districts of Iglesias in the southwest and Sarrabus in the southeast. Mining had powerful incentives — the favoring legislation of the Liberal regime that ended the monopoly of the Crown over the subsoil and opened it to exploration and extraction; the growing demand for raw materials from the growth of industry on the mainland; and the transport revolution that made continental markets accessible. The industry therefore expanded exponentially in the closing decades of the century. The output of the mining industry as measured in tons quintupled between 1860 and 1900, and the workforce tripled from 5,000 to 15,000. It was the misfortune of the miners that mosquitoes bred in the damp mine shafts, and that poverty, a deficient diet, and substandard housing were powerful risk factors for the disease. By 1900, malaria had become the most important health concern among the mining population. The great mining center of Montevarchi, where malaria dominated all other causes of admission to the infirmary and where 70 per cent of miners reported in 1902 that they had suffered from the disease in the previous year.

Along with the immediate circumstances that followed in the wake of deforestation and the development of mining, Sardinia in the late nineteenth century offered a host of social conditions that favored malaria, which thrives on human misfortune. The population of the island consisted principally of impoverished peasants who performed outdoor manual labor at the height of the malaria season in the valleys and coastal plains where anophelines were most abundant. The peasants lived in housing that was porous and open to flying insects; their immune systems were compromised by under- and malnutrition; they were inadequately protected by deficient clothing; and they were unable to defend themselves because of pervasive illiteracy and sanitary ignorance. The symbiotic relationship between malaria and poverty was well known to health officials on the island. The eminent physician Giuseppe Zagari, for example, stressed that all Sardinians bore the stigmata of chronic malaria — emaciation and a painful swelling of the spleen — on their bodies. But the poor whom he identified as those who lived on a diet of beans, corn meal, and snails suffered the complications and sequelae of the disease far more than their more well fed neighbors, and they had the highest incidence of the extreme neurological deficit caused by malaria known as cachexia.

Economic circumstances promoting indigence were therefore a further factor that directly undermined the health of southern Italian peasants in general and of Sardinians in particular. The integration of the region into a national and then international market through unification and modern means of transport meant that the backward, undercapitalized agriculture of the South found itself unable to compete with the advanced and efficient producers of the North of Italy, the Midwest of the United States, and the black earth areas of Russia. Prices for grain products plummeted, rural unemployment soared, and malnutrition prevailed. The effects of this agricultural crisis, which struck hardest between 1880 and 1895, included growing inequality between a relatively advantaged North and an economically backward South, leading to the emergence of the "Southern Question" in Italian history as the expression of the grievances of southerners. In much of the South, including Sardinia, malaria became a leading expression of this sectional issue. Indeed, malaria became the leading public health problem of southern

Italians, especially in Sardinia, which by the turn of the century had earned an unhappy reputation as the most malarious of all Italian regions. Indeed, it was a common saying that every Sardinian had a swollen belly and that the words Sardinia and malaria were synonymous.[16] Malaria, long endemic, had become an emergency.

The First Campaign against Malaria: Before DDT

In part because malaria was the leading public health problem in Italy, causing as many as 100,000 deaths per year at the close of the century, malariology as a discipline emerged as the pride of Italian medical science. It was Italian scientists who played the leading role in unraveling the secrets of the disease, and the so-called "Italian School" of malariology led by such figures as Camillo Golgi, Angelo Celli, and Giovanni Battista Grassi led the field internationally. Above all, the discovery and demonstration of the mosquito theory of transmission by Grassi and Celli after 1898 combined with the sudden new availability of quinine on the international market to suggest the idea of a campaign to eradicate malaria from the nation. Other spurs to action were also at work — a new understanding of the economic, human, and social costs of the disease to the nation; the conviction that there was suddenly a powerful tool to attack the disease; and the pressure of enlightened landlords, mine owners, and railroad entrepreneurs whose businesses were compromised by an ill and unproductive work force.

Thus encouraged to act, the Italian parliament passed a series of measures between 1900 and 1907 that launched an unprecedented national campaign to eradicate malaria by means of the "magic bullet" of quinine — a campaign that was pursued resolutely until 1962, when victory was declared and the entire nation was pronounced malaria-free. At the outset, the strategy was to make use of the now abundant supplies of quinine to medicate the entire population at risk from malaria for several malaria seasons. Since quinine kills plasmodia in the blood stream, the idea was to distribute tablets manufactured by the state both prophylactically and therapeutically with the goal of breaking the chain of transmission. Prophylactically administered, quinine would prevent people from contracting the disease after being bitten by infected mosquitoes. At the same time, quinine used therapeutically would "sterilize" the blood of infected patients, thereby protecting mosquitoes when they took their blood meals. Thus defended against plasmodia by a protective chemical barrier, neither mosquitoes nor humans would be infected, and transmission would cease. The most optimistic members of the

---

[16] "Mosquito Eradication and Malaria Control," excerpt from Trustees' confidential report, 1 January 1954, RAC, Record Group 1.2, Series 700 Europe, box. 12, folder 101.

Italian school, including Grassi, expected their method to yield victory within a few years.

However elegant and simple in theory, the quinine strategy proved ineffective in practice as a stand-alone antimalarial methodology. It was impossible to administer medication to a remote and isolated rural population without making medical care readily accessible. In order to implement the quininization of the entire population, the campaign created a new institution — the rural health station — that became the sheet anchor of the new initiative. The Sardinian provinces of Cagliari and Sassari, for example, were dotted with health stations staffed with physicians, medical students, and nurses from the mainland who provided care, quinine, and health education.

The quinine regimen, however, is lengthy and complicated, and it requires faithful daily compliance. This compliance could not be expected from an illiterate population that had no understanding of the mechanisms of the disease and the necessity for such disciplined observance. Led by Angelo Celli, the founders of the eradication campaign rapidly drew this lesson and urged that education was no less important as an antimalarial than quinine. The result was that the rural health station was soon flanked by a second institution. This was the rural school that, beginning in the Roman Campagna and then spreading across the whole nation, tackled the gigantic problem of illiteracy among both children and adults with a special stress on promoting a "health consciousness" and knowledge of the fundamentals of malaria as a disease.

Thus as it progressed, the campaign adjusted course and moved far from its original narrow focus on a single magic bullet to give attention to a whole range of "social determinants" of disease. In the early years, additional antimalarial measures included access to care and education. In time the campaign created other institutions such as malaria sanatoria and summer camps for children to remove them from the zones of greatest risk and provide them with a sound diet, clothing, and instruction in the fundamentals of the disease. The campaign also turned its attention to labor legislation; wages; housing; land drainage; and environmental sanitation, including the tactic pioneered in Sardinia by Claudio Fermi in the 1920s and 1930s known as *piccola bonifica* — the control and removal of small collections of water on farmsteads.[17]

The passage from the Liberal regime to the Fascist dictatorship after Mussolini's seizure of power in October 1922 marked, in theory, a transformation of the antimalarial campaign. Viewing the persistence of malaria as a symptom of the failure of the Liberal state, Fascism made the defeat of malaria a test of its legitimacy and a centerpiece of its political propaganda. To Fascists, the preceding regime was

---

[17] Fermi, Claudio, *Regioni malariche: decadenza, risanamento e spesa: Sardegna*, 1934, 2 vols.: Rome.

weak and indecisive like all parliamentary democracies, and totalitarianism alone possessed the singleness of will to carry the project through to victory. Referring to Liberal Italy as "petty-minded and flabby," the eminent medical authority and expert on Sardinia Achille Sclavo assured his audience in 1925 that Fascism alone would fulfill the promises of the Liberal state to Sardinia.[18] The new regime, it was claimed, replaced the indecisiveness of democracy with the all-conquering will of a single man. The Duce would rid Italy of malaria, the shameful symbol of Italian backwardness and an enduring threat to weaken the "race" and derail the fascist quest for greatness. Furthermore, in the preparation for a new Roman empire Sardinia had a special place. As the only region in Italy that could plausibly be described in the 1920s as still underpopulated, a medically redeemed Sardinia could serve as a first step in the Fascist vision of imperial expansion. Italy's second largest island could absorb some of the excess population that the regime's pronatalist policies would generate on the mainland. Populating Sardinia with an inflow of settlers and eradicating malaria were two facets of a single project.

Despite the bombast of Fascist rhetoric, the substance of antimalarial policy changed far less than the language used to justify it, the purposes it was intended to serve, and the names of the institutions created to implement it. The characteristically Fascist approach to malaria was to attack it through an integrated program of land reclamation, settlement, and intensification of agriculture known as *bonifica integrale*. In practice, the approach of *bonifica integrale* required such a gigantic commitment of planning and resources in competition with other political and military priorities that it was never seriously implemented on the national level. The two areas of Italy where conditions of extensive marshland and low population density most clearly fit the strategy of *bonifica integrale* were the Pontine Marshes and Sardinia. The Pontine Marshes, which were the showcase of Fascist domestic policy, were the great success of the integrated Fascist approach. Sardinia, where vested interests, expense, and bureaucratic inertia triumphed, was its great failure.

On the eve of the Second World War the Pontine Marshes had been successfully drained, the land settled, and malaria largely controlled. Sardinia, by contrast, had islands of drainage and modernization and a scattering of "new cities," but the island as a whole was still characterized by environmental degradation, an unregulated hydrology, backward agriculture, and pervasive malaria. Furthermore, in relative terms, Sardinia had regressed because, even as the disease declined in absolute terms, the island consolidated its position as the most afflicted of all Italian regions.[19]

---

[18] Tognotti, *Per una storia, op. cit.,* 230–1.

[19] On *bonifica integrale* in the Pontine Marshes, see my work, *The Conquest of Malaria,* chapter 6; and for fascist antimalarial activity in Sardinia, see Tognotti, *Per una storia, op. cit.,* 230–61.

In practice, therefore, if not in theory and in propaganda, the antimalarial campaign of the Fascist era marked a continued application of the tools and the slow patient work that had been pioneered in the Liberal era — quinine distribution, rural health stations, rural schools, and localized environmental sanitation. Other methodologies were taken up and applied selectively — antilarval attacks by means of spraying with Paris Green and gambusia fish, and bonification. Progress continued, but incrementally rather than in a manner consistent with the loudly proclaimed "fascist revolution," and the bases for these advances were the scientific discoveries and public health programs set up before the First World War.

Unfortunately, statistics on the progress of the Italian campaign against malaria are notoriously unreliable, and nowhere more so than in Sardinia. Remote areas and poor means of communication, severe problems of access to medical attention, the shortage of laboratory facilities, and the protean nature of the symptomatology of malaria itself that enables it to mimic other diseases — all of these factors meant that an accurate statistical profile of the disease prior to the intensive scrutiny of the Sardinian Project is impossible. Data for mortality, in any case, were more reliable than those for morbidity. Nevertheless, there is a consensus that significant progress was achieved throughout Italy, and on the island. Official, though highly approximate, comparative statistics for average annual mortality from "malarial fever and swamp cachexia" per 100,000 inhabitants clearly illustrate the severity of the disease and the "sad primacy" of Sardinia among all Italian regions at the start of the campaign, and the striking progress achieved by the early and late 1930s. The figures are indicated in Table 1.1.[20]

A practical consequence of the reliance on quinine was that the decline of mortality during this period was more dramatic than the decline in morbidity. The availability of the antiplasmodial, in other words, meant that cases could be treated and death prevented even though transmission continued. The downturn in malaria incidence was significantly slower than the drop in mortality.

The Crisis after World War II

The advance in the control of malaria was not an unbroken, linear progression. On the contrary, the severity of the annual summer epidemic varied from year to year according to the vicissitudes of the weather pattern. Years of abundant rainfall lasting late into the spring together with high summer temperatures were the delight of anopheline mosquitoes. The most severe and lasting setbacks, however, were the results of war. The first and second world wars both reversed the gains of decades of patient effort and left dramatic malaria epidemics in their wake.

---

[20] Tognotti, *Per una storia, op.cit.*, 76, 252.

Table 1.1: Average Annual Malaria Mortality Per 100,000 Inhabitants.

Region	1900–1913	1929–1934	1935–1939
Piedmont	3.5	0.2	0.2
Veneto	7.4	0.3	0.3
Liguria	0.9	0.5	0.2
Lombardy	4.8	2.4	0.5
Emilia	7.5	0..5	0.3
Tuscany	9.5	1.2	0.4
Marches	2.2	0.7	0.1
Umbria	3.9	0.6	0.3
Lazio	42.0	8.1	1.3
Abruzzi	41.5	4.9	1.2
Campania	26.5	4.1	1.5
Apulia	134.0	23.2	5.2
Basilicata	183.7	38.9	10.0
Calabria	104.7	20.8	8.7
Sicily	97.7	11.6	5.4
Sardinia	211.2	43.5	20.7
Italy	40.3	6.4	2.2

The reasons behind the public health calamity that followed the wars of both the Liberal and the Fascist regimes are multiple and interlocking because malaria as a disease thrives on human misfortune. Warfare effectively brought the antimalarial campaign to a halt as medical personnel were conscripted and diverted from civilian to military needs, and as the collapse of the international supply of quinine deprived the movement of its chief tool.

A second cascade of public health consequences followed from the impact of war on the two mainstays of the Sardinian economy — agriculture and mining. With regard to agriculture, the world wars involved a systematic diversion of resources from the countryside to industry and the military. Draft animals and machinery were requisitioned; manpower was drafted; fertilizers, parts, fuel, and equipment became unavailable; investment ceased; land drainage projects were halted; and non-immune women and children replaced absent men in the fields. But agricultural machinery and draft animals were themselves coefficients of health, and their disappearance increased the numbers of people exposed to infection in the fields and reduced the alternative sources of blood meals apart from man available to flying insects. Furthermore, with shortages of every kind, soil was eroded, and production declined sharply while the infrastructure of irrigation and drainage systems was neglected. The collapse of the transportation system of boats, trains, motor vehicles, and horse-drawn carts disrupted distribution networks so that food shortages developed even when supply was adequate. Prices rose remorselessly, and the problems worsened dramatically under the influence of hoarding and black marketeering. Throughout the mining districts as well, the impact of the conflict was devastating. With supplies, equipment, and transport all unavailable, it became impossible to maintain the shafts, which flooded and were closed. The industry, the prefect of Cagliari reported, was reduced to a state of "total paralysis," and the workers were dismissed en masse. [21] American officials, forgetting that the Sardinian miners' immediate problem was the absence of work, tellingly if somewhat confusing described their living conditions as those of slave labor.[22]

Military action of course contributed to the epidemic crisis. The mobilization of large numbers of young men, some of them lacking all immunity, and their deployment under crowded and unsanitary conditions in malarial zones both in Italy and in the Balkans exposed them to infection. The stationing in Sardinia of 200,000 troops who were cut off from the mainland after the fall of Mussolini in July 1943 and who therefore lacked logistical support, food supplies, and medicine complicated the public health and food emergencies. The soldiers of the Savoy Division, which was stationed in highly malarial zones of Cagliari province, suffered extensively from malaria.[23] The consequences of Mussolini's military adventures devastated health. Defeat, occupation, the disintegration of the army after September 8, 1943, and the transformation of the peninsula into a war zone further decimated agriculture, industry, and the transport system; produced large numbers of displaced and homeless people; and subjected the occupied nation to the German policy of viewing Italy as place to be pillaged for raw materials, industrial plant, and labor. A series of Allied bombing raids on Sardinia from February 1943 also caused extensive destruction and unleashed floods of refugees who sheltered in improvised and overcrowded accommodations. These were all factors destructive of resistance to disease.

The situation confronting ERLAAS at the outset of its Project at the end of 1945 was dramatic, with the agricultural sector further crippled in 1945 by the

---

[21] Prefect of Cagliari, Relazione sull'attività politico-economica relativa al mese di maggio 1945, n. 1781.Archivio Centrale dello Stato (ACS), Direzione Generale della Pubblica Sicurezza (PS), 1944–1946, b. 17, fasc. 14 (Cagliari).

[22] Meeting Re Relief for Carbonia Held in Mr.Keeny's Office, 5 October 1945, United Nations Archives (UNA), UNRRA, 1943–1949, PAG – 4/3.0.14.0.0.2.:1.

[23] Tognotti, *Per una storia, op.cit.,* 262.

worst drought ever recorded on the island with no rainfall between January 29 and the end of the year.[24] Unhappily, 1946 was also exceptionally dry.[25] Yields per acre for nearly every crop were a fraction of prewar levels, and vast areas were left unplanted, as the soil was too hard and dry for plowing or planting. Fodder crops failed as well, so that animal husbandry collapsed as farm animals were slaughtered or faced starvation, while the oxen that survived were too lean to drag the plow.[26] Forest fires blazed across the landscape, destroying orchards, vineyards, and crops in their path.[27] There were almost Biblical plagues of locusts and grasshoppers.[28] Inflation was an inevitable result as consumers were caught in a scissors crisis between wages for a manual laborer that increased ninefold over prewar levels and prices that increased twenty-fold.[29] The island faced hunger, and even state rations could raise the daily caloric intake of the average Sardinian to only 900 calories per day of the 2,600 considered necessary for health. A typical family in the crisis years of 1945–1946 spent 90% of its income on food.[30] Faced with empty shops and no money, the population also dressed in rags and either went barefoot or wore shoes that were falling to pieces. According to American experts, the "outstanding facts" in 1945–1946 were that "prices of the necessities of life are increasing much more rapidly than wages", leading to "hardship and a declining standard of living."[31] This declining standard found clear expression in a crisis of public health. Although malaria and tuberculosis were by far the greatest concerns, the authorities also faced serious outbreaks of other diseases — trachoma, syphilis, and gastroenteritis among adults and scabies, vitamin deficiencies, and pertussis among children.[32]

---

[24] Prefect of Cagliari, Relazione sull'attività politico economica relativa al mese di agosto 1945, n. 3064.ACS, PS, 1944–1946, b. 17, fasc. 14 (Cagliari).

[25] UNRRA: Sardinia Region, Monthly Report for Period August 19 - September 18, 1946., UNA, UNRRA, 3.0.14.2.0, Box 31.

[26] Prefect of Cagliari, Relazione mensile sulla situazione della provincia per il mese di dicembre 1945, 31 Dec. 1945, n. 5781. ACS, PS, 1944–1946, b. 17, fasc. 14 (Cagliari).

[27] UNRRA: Sardinia Region, Monthly Report for Period August 19 - September 18, 1946., UNA, UNRRA, 3.0.14.2.0, Box 31.

[28] "Notes on the Use of Gammexane in Sardinia in 1946," UNA, UNRRA, 3.0.14.2.0, Box 24, Folder RD/15/12; and Silvio Sirigu, Press Digest: UNRRA Assistance to Sardinia from *Il Nuovo Giornale d'Italia*," 12 December 1946. UNA, UNRRA, 1943–1949, PAG 4/3.0.14.0.0.2:1.

[29] Edward L. Sard, Italian Relief and Rehabilitation Needs, 10 November 1945; and William G. Wolk, Notes on Economic Reporting — Brief Summary of the Italian Economy, 24 November 1945. UNA, UNRRA , 3.0.14.0.0.1, Box 2, folder "Mr.Sard".

[30] Harran Cleveland, Speech of 27 September 1946. UNA, UNRRA, 4/3.0.14.0.0.2:1.

[31] Wolk, *op. cit.,* 62.

[32] Prefect of Cagliari, Relazione sull'attività politico-economica relativa al mese di maggio 1945, n. 1781.ACS, PS 1944-1946, b. 17, fasc. 14 (Cagliari).

A crime wave also swept over Sardinia. War veterans, ex-partisans, prisoners of war, and forced laborers in Germany returned to the island to face unemployment and starvation. They joined with unemployed farm workers and escaped prisoners to form marauding bands armed with hand grenades, rifles, and submachine guns diverted from the war effort. These bands carried out robbery, kidnapping, extortion, and murder while the undermanned police forces, disrupted and demoralized by occupation and a change of regime, struggled to re-establish authority. At the same time speculators, hoarders, and black marketers enriched themselves and embittered hardship with their predations. The police reported despair and hunger; a flood of beggars; a great surge in prostitution, especially of minors; and a "moral crisis of society." [33]

The Second Campaign against Malaria: ERLAAS and DDT

American policies towards Sardinia, as for Italy as a whole, evolved as the full extent of the social, economic, and medical disaster emerged. The first task, however, was to prevent a public health disaster from epidemic diseases that threatened to cause immense suffering, to unravel the economy, and to complicate the task of restoring stable government. Typhus, typhoid, and tuberculosis all caused concern and sparked intervention, but the overwhelming threat was that of malaria. The instrument to eradicate the threat of malaria — ERLAAS — therefore managed the greatest public health program of the postwar era.

ERLAAS, however, needs to be seen in a political as well as a public health context. As the decision to deploy DDT was being made, the Cold War was unfolding, and the war against *Anopheles labranchiae* reflected the logic of the conflict of the West against communism. The Rockefeller Foundation, which directed ERLAAS and provided its strategic thinking, was motivated by a humanitarian concern to promote health by supporting medical research and campaigns against selected infectious diseases. At the same time it was fully aware that medicine, science, and public health were not simply means to relieve suffering, but also instruments of "soft power" to promote American

---

[33] Prefect of Cagliari, Relazione sull'attività politico-economica relativa al mese di giugno 1945, 2 July 1945, n.2175. ACS, PS, 1944–1946, b. 17, fasc. 14 (Cagliari); Direzione Generale della Pubblica Sicurezza, Sardegna — sicurezza pubblica, 30 April 1946, n. 555/290. ACS, PS, 1944, b. 123; and, Direzione Generale P.S., Situazione Politica, ordine pubblico, situazione economico-annonaria, spirito pubblico, condizioni della pubblica sicurezza nelle provincie tornate all'amministrazione italiana [Lazio (Roma-Frosinone-Littoria), Abruzzi (Campobasso), Campania, Puglia, Lucania, Calabria, Sicilia, Sardegna] nel mese di agosto 1944. ACS, PS 1944–1946, b. 14, fasc. 2 (agosto 1944).

hegemony.[34] Defeating malaria by means of DDT first in Sardinia and then on a global level would provide a stunning display of the power of American science and technology. Enlightened self-interest also indicated that a postwar global market economy required healthy consumers and producers, and that an inexpensive and rapid means of achieving health would pay lasting dividends, and all the more so if American firms such as Du Pont and Monsanto played a prominent role in supplying the hydrocarbon. Furthermore, the "American solution" to the problem of malaria would obviate the need to attend to the social determinants of disease such as poverty, inequality, and environmental degradation by social and economic measures that smacked of social medicine and even of socialism.

The ERLAAS approach, devised in the fall of 1945 and first implemented in 1946/1947, relied heavily on a military approach to the problem. The organization employed military terms and metaphors in its internal documents, it followed strict principles of hierarchy and control, and it made use of military equipment in its work.[35] This "second Normandy landing" and the quasi military occupation of the island that followed took no notice of the history of the island, of the living conditions of the population, of the Sardinian economy, or even of the prior record of the antimalarial campaign that had begun in 1900. Instead, the planners drew up a map of Sardinia and divided it up into a hierarchical series of administrative divisions — regions, divisions, sections, districts, and sectors — with the sector as the most important operational unit, defined as the area that a single spraying team could treat with DDT in a day. For each of the 5,299 sectors the mappers employed scouts to conduct a survey of every manmade structure within the sector where *Anopheles labranchiae* could rest — houses, mine shafts, public buildings, churches, stores, barns, bridges, pig-sties, stables, sheds, chicken-houses, culverts, and the ancient towers known as *nuraghi* that are a feature of the Sardinian landscape. Caves and grottoes were also designated for treatment. Having thus defined and identified the task, the ERLAAS administrators recruited teams of sprayers from the local population of peasants, farm workers, and laborers who would have detailed knowledge of the geography of the area. One team was employed for each sector, and equipped with hand and shoulder sprayers, canisters of 5%

[34] The term is that of Joseph S. Nye, *Soft Power: The Means to Success in World Politics*, Public Affairs, 2004: New York.

[35] The military nature of the Sardinian Project and the expression "Normandy landing" are stressed by Eugenia Tognotti, Program to eradicate malaria in Sardinia, 1946–1950, *Emerging Infectious Diseases* Sept. 2009, **15**(9), available from http://www.cdc.gov/EID/content/15/9/1460.htm. Consulted on August 21, 2010.

DDT solution suspended in oil, and the transport needed to reach and traverse the sector — Jeeps, mules, or, most frequently, boots. Their instructions were to cover the walls and ceilings of each structure with a film of DDT at the rate of 2 grams per square meter that would not only kill mosquitoes on contact but would also last with a lethal residual effect that would destroy insects for months until the subsequent spraying.

This original strategy was based on the unprecedented killing power of DDT and on the assumption that *A. labranchiae* was highly endophilic, spending most of its time nestling indoors before and between blood meals. The goal, then, was to poison all resting places in the malarial off-season between November and February so that overwintering anophelines would be destroyed and few would emerge in the spring to breed and re-establish the cycle of transmission. A further refinement was that, at the completion of each week of spraying throughout a district, the scouts would return to verify that the spray application had been carried out to specification, and to find and count mosquitoes. The directors of the Project, eventually gathering in a "war room" in Cagliari, collected the information, projected it onto maps of the island, and planned the succeeding campaign. They also awarded prizes for successful spraying and scouting, punished slackers, and fostered a spirit of competition between the teams.

Entomological evidence revealed, however, that the habits of *A. labranchiae* were not so domestic as the original design of the Project had envisaged. Instead of sheltering solely in man-made structures, the Sardinian vector was largely sylvatic, resting out-of-doors and entering dwellings chiefly for the purpose of feeding after dark. As a result, the idea of eradicating the species by means of residual interior spraying was problematic.[36] Therefore, from 1947, ERLAAS reduced indoor spraying to secondary importance in the campaign, and instead stressed the strategy of spraying outdoor breeding places in the spring and summer in line with the curve of cases that first appeared in May, climbed steeply in June and July, and then peaked in August before fading away in November after a possible secondary spike in October in years with a rainy September.[37] The sprayers followed a technique of climatic zoning according to altitude. The squads began their work at sea level in March when anophelines first bred along the coast and then the teams worked their way progressively onto higher elevations as warm weather advanced.

---

[36] Logan, *The Sardinian Project, op. cit.*, 66.

[37] As Logan wrote, "It was believed that.... eradication depended on larviciding and that although residual treatment undoubtedly helped, its effect was not conclusive and the time and money involved could be better spent in larviciding." *The Sardinian Project, op. cit.*, 44; 67.

The administrative divisions of the projects and the reliance on teams of sprayers and scouts persisted, but the thrust of the program turned from adult mosquitoes to larvae and from human structures to mountain pools, puddles in river beds, the edges of streams, marshes, lakes, irrigation ditches, and wells.

Outdoor spraying was a far more labor-intensive task than residual indoor spraying. The spray, consisting of a 5% solution of DDT in diesel oil, had to be renewed on a weekly basis throughout the breeding season. Furthermore, there were over a million breeding sites, and of these many were hidden beneath thick covers of vegetation and brambles. The spraying itself, often had to be preceded by the draining of marshes; stream clearance; dynamiting; and the rectification of river beds to increase their flow. Outdoor spraying, therefore, required an array of equipment that was not needed for indoor applications — brush hooks, axes, shovels, picks, scythes, boats, rafts, tractors, ditchers, mowers, pumps, and explosives. In addition, some expanses of water were so extensive that they could not be effectively treated by hand, and were sprayed instead by pilots from the Italian air force flying converted bombers with fuel drums in place of weaponry under their wings. There was also the problem that shepherds and fisherman, fearing that the application of DDT would kill the sheep and fish on which they depended, hid water collections from the work teams and occasionally opened fire on them with their rifles. Bandits attacked ERLAAS payroll deliveries, and communists denounced the entire program as an assertion of American power over the region.[38] Faced with such obstacles and with such an arduous task stretching across thousands of square miles of inaccessible and rugged terrain, ERLAAS found itself compelled to hire a virtual army of workers, numbering as many as 30,000 at the high point of the effort, with 24,000 engaged in the heavy manual labor of draining and clearing rather than spraying itself.[39]

Thus configured, the Sardinian Project reached its peak in the years 1947–1948 with full-scale spraying underway throughout the island both indoors and outdoors. 1948/1949 marked a turning point. Scouts reported large swathes of territory that exhibited both "larval negativity" outdoors and "adult negativity" indoors. The emphasis shifted in 1949, therefore, from all-out spraying to mopping up sectors where the scouts had found indications of positivity for *A. labranchiae*. By 1951 the numbers of mosquitoes of all species had been severely decimated, but here and there *A. labranchiae* persisted. Since the initial objective of the Project had been to determine the feasibility of eradicating an indigenous mosquito species, the campaign was technically a failure. From the

[38] Tognotti, Americani, comunisti e zanzare *op. cit.,;* Logan, *The Sardinian Project, op. cit.,* 44.
[39] Logan, *The Sardinian Project, op. cit.,*44–5.

Table 1.2: Officially Reported Cases of Malaria Per Annum.

Year	Cases
1946	75,447
1947	39,303
1948	15,121
1949	1,314
1950	40
1951	9

standpoint of public health, however, the chain of transmission had been broken, Sardinia was malaria-free, and the Project ceased. In the words of the Rockefeller Foundation,

At the end of the effort it was still possible to find an occasional *Anopheles labranchiae* mosquito — and so one could not say that the campaign for eradication had been successful. The experiment demonstrated that an indigenous insect is more difficult to exterminate than a species that is lately come to the environment. But while the answer to the eradication question was negative, the results of the experiment in terms of public health advancement were rewardingly affirmative.[40]

The numbers of officially reported cases followed the downward trajectory of Table 1.2.[41]

Logan, noting that the Project had attracted "world-wide interest," predicted confidently as early as 1948 that it "will point the way to an eradication technique applicable on a large scale, heretofore impossible."[42]

Additional Factors in Eradication

There is a consensus that DDT was a potent factor in the successful eradication of malaria from Sardinia, but the conclusion that it acted as a stand-alone instrument is deeply misleading. The postwar spraying took place in the midst of a series of

---

[40] "Mosquito Eradication and Malaria Control," excerpt from Trustees' confidential report, January 1, 1954. RAC, Record Group 1.2, Series 700 Europe, box. 12, folder 101, 17.

[41] *Ibid.*

[42] Letter of John A. Logan, Sardinia *Anopheles* Eradication Project, August 1948, RAC, Record Group 1.2, Series 700 Europe, Folder 113, box 13.

overlapping interventions unrelated to DDT that are not mentioned in Logan's official account or subsequent histories of the Project. One factor that is all too readily overlooked is that the establishment of ERLAAS itself had a transformative impact on the Sardinian labor market. Once the antimalarial organization had shifted to a policy of outdoor spraying, it rapidly became the largest employer on the island, hiring as many as 30,000 workers at rates higher than government wages for a five-year period of campaigning. ERLAAS thereby made a significant contribution to combating poverty and unemployment — two of the principal social preconditions to the vulnerability of Sardinians to malaria. The final total of US $11,000,000 that it spent on the island — a sum far in excess of original estimates — also stimulated the regional economy. In that sense the implementation of the DDT program silently introduced a second important variable into the experiment, and the trustees of the Rockefeller Foundation even noted that Project expenditures marked the "economic rehabilitation" of the island.[43]

Furthermore, even Paul Russell, the proponent of the "DDT era of malariology," noted that the spraying itself introduced a further variable into the experiment. In his view, the "Sardinia Project" initiated a progressive upward spiral in which mosquito reduction and agricultural improvement mutually reinforced one another. The spraying program, he wrote in 1949 while it was still in progress, had already produced "collateral benefits to Sardinia." Peasants were able to "open up new lands for agriculture" and to "go ahead with bonifica projects formerly impossible because of malaria."[44]

But there is more to it than that. The records of ERLAAS and of the Rockefeller Foundation make no acknowledgement of the long history of patient antimalarial work on the island over the half century before the launching of the Project. The impression is that the American intervention began from nothing. There is an in-built institutional bias in the documentation towards proving that the "American" technological approach to malaria eradication by DDT alone was effective. In fact, however, ERLAAS owed much of its success to the fact that the ground had been prepared in advance for its activities. A major example is the ease with which the sprayers carried out their work. They encountered scattered opposition from bandits, shepherds, and communists. In general, however, the documents of the Project make it clear that the overwhelming majority of Sardinians welcomed the ERLAAS men onto their fields and into their homes. This enthusiastic reception marks a striking contrast to the widespread antagonism encountered early in the

---

[43] "Mosquito eradication and Malaria Control," excerpt from Trustees' confidential report, January 1, 1954. RAC, Record Group 1.2, Series 700 Europe, box. 12, folder 101, 15–17.

[44] RAC, Record Group 1.2, Series 700 Europe, box 14, folder 116. Letter of Paul Russell to Alberto Missiroli, 3 Nov. 1949.

century when physicians and public health officials began to distribute quinine capsules. At that time, the antimalarial campaigners stress the popular suspicion that the medicine was a poison and part of a nefarious plot by the state to solve the problem of poverty by settling scores with the poor. The health of Sardinians was so compromised and fevers so familiar that peasants and workers often were unaware of the specific importance of malaria. Just as in the time of Alessandro Manzoni and Giovanni Verga, the countryside teemed with rumors of poisoners (*untori*) and of a great diabolical plot.

Thus, one of the greatest initial difficulties of the first campaign was stubborn resistance by those most in need of its benefits. Peasants, farm workers, miners, and shepherds refused to attend the newly opened clinics. They barricaded themselves in their homes and turned away visiting physicians and nurses. Alternatively, they accepted the suspect medicine they were offered, but then they hoarded it for later resale or barter for cigarettes; they spat the capsules on the ground after the intruders had departed; or they fed the offending tablets to their pigs. A portion of the subsidized Italian quinine also made its way to the black market, where it was re-exported to meet the demand of malarial areas of North Africa, where Italian state quinine commanded a high price because of its guaranteed purity. Sometimes parents cautiously swallowed their own medicine, but adamantly refused to administer it to their children. Most commonly of all, patients who were seriously ill took quinine just long enough to suppress their fever, after which they ignored the remainder of the required regimen. Thus, public health officials estimated in 1909 that the majority of the quinine distributed was not consumed.[45]

This suspicion and ignorance greatly complicated the work of the campaign, and a major effort was devoted to finding ways to overcome it. These included education, sermons advocating quinine, health stations that offered a full range of services in order to gain the trust of patients, and public health displays in which villages notables demonstrated their confidence by publicly swallowing the medication. In this way, the tireless campaign between 1900 and the establishment of ERLAAS in 1945 promoted a public health consciousness that was the backdrop to the enthusiasm that greeted the sprayers. Quinine, in a sense, had prepared Sardinians to understand the necessity for DDT.

Even the ability of the Sardinian Project to deploy scouts and sprayers so effectively depended on the fact that the recruiters could count on their workers already possessing some understanding of the rudiments of malaria transmission and of the importance of their work. Marston Bates, one of the leading Rockefeller men, revealed more than he realized when he wrote that, "Eradication is possible, but

---

[45] ACS, PS (1882–1915), b. 124, fasc. Chinino di Stato: affari generali. Ispettore Generale Medico Ravicini, Appunto per l'Illmo Signor Direttore Generale della Sanità Pubblica, 15 May 1909.

requires a tightly organized and smooth functioning administrative machine."[46] Such a machine could emerge and run smoothly only if the island possessed abundant personnel educated in the essentials of malaria as a disease to staff it.

It is suggestive that ERLAAS itself built on the legacy of decades by carrying out an educational mission of its own. It offered weekly lessons in Grassi's "doctrine" of mosquito transmission to its personnel; it provided the schools of Sardinia with a syllabus on which to base lessons for all the children of the island; it broadcasted radio programs on malaria and the mission to eradicate it; and it printed leaflets, posters, and bulletins for distribution across the region.[47]

Thus, the performance of the Sardinian Project is misconstrued if one ignores the long history of antimalarial work on the island that smoothed the way for the postwar campaign. In addition, however, the history of ERLAAS is distorted by confining attention to the records and archives pertaining to the DDT experiment. The reason is that those materials, like John Logan's official account, deal with the Sardinian Project as if it had proceeded in isolation, ignoring the array of initiatives undertaken by authorities other than ERLAAS. Those initiatives had purposes that were ostensibly non-medical but that nevertheless had a major impact on the vulnerability of the population to malaria. The Sardinian Project is therefore best understood in a broader context of efforts to confront the social and economic as well as the medical dimensions of the crisis.

The most important intervention operating simultaneously with the Sardinian Project was that of UNRRA (United Nations Relief and Rehabilitation Administration), which functioned in Italy with overwhelmingly American funding from 1945 to 1947, and was succeeded by the Marshall Plan. Like the Sardinian Project, UNRRA and Marshall aid combined humanitarian intentions and Cold War priorities. In terms of the Sardinian Project, UNRRA was the decisive program because it was more tightly linked with the battle against malaria, and the effects of the Marshall Plan were felt after the decisive battles against *A. labranchiae* had already been won. UNRRA helped the Project to achieve victory, and the Marshall Plan consolidated the triumph.

UNRRA's objectives in Italy were both long- and short-term. "Relief" was the immediate aim, and it entailed combating the twin evils of "disorder" and "disease." "Disorder" signified strikes, demonstrations, riots, advances in the strength of the Italian socialist and communist parties, and any degree of economic hardship that would drive workers and peasants into supporting left-wing trade unions

---

[46] RAC, Record Group 1.2, Series 700 Europe, box 13, folder 114. Letter of Marston Bates to G.K. Strode, 23 May 1949.

[47] RAC, Record Group 1.2, Series 700 Europe, box 13, folder 113. C. Garrett-Jones, *Anopheles Eradication in Sardinia*, 23 March 1949, 10.

and political parties. The task was at once a humanitarian "international responsibility" and a "form of world insurance" against revolution.

The first priorities in combating disorder were to alleviate hunger and to contain inflation, and the thinking of American planners was that both goals could be achieved by the massive importation and distribution of the necessities needed to keep Italian families in health. The means were the "three ships a day policy" by which three ships bearing American goods docked daily at Italian ports and unloaded urgently needed supplies, with each ship representing 550 Italian railroad cars of material. These supplies were transported in turn by train and truck to each of the eight regions into which Italy had been divided, and of which Sardinia was one. After the supplies arrived in specific communes, they were distributed to needy people in the locality by committees consisting of local notables — the mayor, parish priests, doctors, school teachers, businessmen, and other authorities — whose standing and legitimacy would also be enhanced by the largesse. The supplies made available to hungry Sardinians included flour, powdered milk, lard, vegetables, semolina, sugar, and canned fish.[48] Clearly food supplies and the control of inflation had important implications not just for political stability and the relief of suffering but also for the enhancement of the population's resistance to disease. Improving the diet and increasing the purchasing power of impoverished Sardinians was a powerful coadjutant to the efforts of the Sardinian Project, coming to the island, it was said, "like oil to a lamp that was dying out."[49]

In addition to dealing indirectly with disease, UNRRA furnished assistance that was immediately linked to the antimalarial efforts on the island. This assistance included hospital and medical supplies, and in particular the synthetic antimalarial quinacrine (Atebrin), which had been synthesized in 1931 and had largely replaced quinine in the immediate postwar armamentarium. Quinine was reserved for intravenous administration for the most serious comatose cases. Along with vector control by DDT, the traditional Italian effort to attack plasmodia in the blood stream recommenced. At the same time, UNRRA funded the establishment of sanatoria in healthy locations for malaria patients and summer camps for children at the seaside and in the mountains. There they could be shielded from biting insects, furnished a sound diet, and educated in the basics of malaria prevention. Pregnant and nursing women were also offered special rations, clothing, and shoes. Concurrent efforts were launched to repair damaged housing, and to provide accommodation for refugees and the displaced. Large numbers of the most

---

[48] A succinct description of the UNRRA distribution program is UNRRA: Italy Mission, Three Ships a Day for Italy: 1946 Program, (n.d.). UNA, UNRRA, 1944–1949, PAG 4/3014001-2:3.

[49] Silvio Sirigu, Press Digest: UNRRA Assistance to Sardinia from *Il Nuovo Giornale d'Italia,* 12 December 1946. UNA, UNRRA, 1943–1949, PAG – 4/3.0.14.0.0.2.:1

vulnerable sectors of the population were thus at least partially protected from infection.

In addition to "relief", the UNRRA mission stressed "rehabilitation," which meant restoring the shattered Italian economy. The goal was to re-establish industry and agriculture to prewar levels of production. Postwar American planners were convinced that the totalitarian regimes of interwar Europe and the Second World War had their roots in the Great Depression and autarchic economic policies. To prevent communism and renewed warfare, the United States therefore offered massive support to restore Italian production and to reintegrate the nation into a global free market economy. In Sardinian terms, this intervention primarily affected agriculture. Peasants and farmers were provided with seeds, fertilizer, fuel, mechanical equipment, and assistance to repair damaged and neglected irrigation and drainage networks. Crops were also sprayed with insecticide to destroy locusts. The results were to increase production, but also to attack malaria indirectly by increasing employment and intensifying agriculture in ways that control water and eliminate mosquito breeding sites.

UNRRA also contributed directly to antimalarial campaigning in Sardinia in two ways. The first was that proceeds of the sale of American goods provided free to the Italian government were used to establish a Lire Fund to finance public health. In Sardinia the Lire Fund was the financial mainstay of ERLAAS. In this way the Sardinian Project is clearly intelligible only in a context that includes the broader relief activities of UNRRA, which financed it. But UNRRA also financed the restoration of the infrastructure of the prewar antimalarial effort, allowing Provincial Antimalarial Committees, health stations, and schools to resume functioning along with the distribution of Atebrin. In this sense the Sardinian Project did not work in isolation at all, but alongside the revival of the antimalarial efforts of the prewar period. Indeed, the traditional antimalarial work began again under American aegis as early as the transmission season of 1944 when the Allied Military Government launched an antimalarial program that its Public Health Division had planned in October 1943 and that continued uninterruptedly alongside the Sardinian Project.[50]

Conclusion

The successful eradication of malaria in Sardinia has significance as a hopeful example of victory over a deadly and incapacitating disease that continues to hold much of the world, and especially sub-Saharan Africa, in its thrall.

---

[50] Russell, Memorandum on Malaria, *op. cit.*, 5–7.

Today, approximately one million people die annually of malaria, which is both treatable and preventable. It remains the most significant tropical disease and, synergistically with HIV/AIDS and tuberculosis, perhaps the world's most serious infectious disease.

It is important, therefore, to draw accurate conclusions from the Sardinian experience — to provide, that is, a historically valid account of the Sardinian Project. The World Health Organization and the international community initially drew an inaccurate lesson from the Sicilian DDT experiment, reaching the logically fallacious conclusion that, because eradication followed DDT spraying, it was caused by DDT spraying.

The reality of the Project is more complex and nuanced. It does of course demonstrate the importance of technological tools, as the role of both Atebrin and, above all, DDT in the final stage of eradication amply confirms. The control of malaria requires ongoing scientific research and the practical use of its results. On the other hand, the antimalarial campaigners who manned the health stations in Sardinia and in rural Italy as a whole learned even before the First World War that the idea of relying on a single scientific weapon was misguided. Malaria, they reported, is the infectious disease that most closely reflects the totality of the relations of human beings with their environment and with one another. Malaria, they argued, is at once a disease of poverty, of environmental degradation, of poor nutrition, of inadequate housing, of illiteracy, of neglect, of population displacement, and of improper agricultural cultivation. The campaign advanced significantly only when free quinine — the first magic bullet — was distributed in a context that included improved housing and wages, literacy, adequate nutrition, and the moral commitment of the political authorities of the nation. These factors were antimalarials of no less importance than quinine itself. Malaria receded with advancing social justice as well as a powerful tool. Even with the most powerful antimalarial technologies, the question remains: what is the appropriate context for their deployment?

Angelo Celli, one of the founders of the antimalarial campaign at the turn of the twentieth century, replied to this question with a motto that has great contemporary relevance — "Do one thing, but do not omit others."[51] As Celli suggested, the lesson of Sardinia may be that an effective antimalarial program should involve a multifaceted initiative. It requires North/South partnership; the moral awakening of affluent powers to the vicious cycle of poverty and disease; education to teach populations how to protect their own health; access to care; affordable treatment; environmental sanitation; and the tools provided by basic scientific research. In

---

[51] B. Fantini, *Unum facere et alterum non omittere*: antimalarial strategies in Italy, 1880–1930, *Parassitologia*, 40(1–2), 1998, esp. 100.

addition, Celli's motto suggests another lesson of Sardinia — the need for malaria control to be based on a long-term commitment and not a "quick fix." Eradication occurred on the island only after half a century of campaigning. Finally, Sardinian success illustrates the importance of large-scale international assistance. Sardinia realized the final goal of eradication with the financial and technical support of the United States and an explicit recognition that disease is an international problem in which the entire community has a vital stake. Malaria is a crisis not of nations but of humanity.

Despite such somber lessons regarding the complexity of eradication, the Sardinian Project also presents a hopeful example of the role that eradication can play in repaying the effort by unleashing the resources of a region. The postwar development of Sardinia in the following decades presupposed the condition that malaria no longer continued to stunt productivity, limit education, consume resources, and enforce poverty. Sardinia today is an illustration of the social, economic, and cultural possibilities that become available when malaria is vanquished.

5 Popular Education and Participation in Malaria Control: A Historical Overview[1]

Socrates Litsios

Introduction

After a long career working for the Rockefeller Foundation as a malariologist, Marshall Barber concluded, in his 1946 autobiography *A Malariologist in Many Lands,* that "a vast proportion of the disease would disappear, almost overnight," if "only one could convince people that mosquitoes carry malaria and teach them a few simple means of protection …. We need not be discouraged," he continued, "if it requires a generation or two among some peoples to accomplish much education..."[2]

Barber, of course, was not the first, nor the last malariologist to highlight the importance of an educated public for malaria control. In fact, much earlier in the 20th century, Italy's approach to malaria, as discussed below, provided an outstanding example of popular education and participation (PEP). Nevertheless, PEP did not become a stable feature of malaria control programs for reasons that are explored in this chapter.

Although PEP has been advocated throughout the last 100 years, the rationale for its importance has changed with the change in technologies available for

[1] An earlier version of this paper was presented at the 2008 Yale conference on the Global Crisis of Malaria. I would like to thank Prof. Frank Snowden for the invitation to address the conference, and Prof. James Webb for his critical comments on my earlier paper, which led to my deciding to radically revise it. Archival research carried out at the Rockefeller Archives Center (RAC) was supported by two RAC grants. I wish to acknowledge with gratitude the assistance provided by Robert Battaly, Assistant Director, Head of Processing, RAC.
[2] M. Barber, *A Malariologist in Many Lands*, University of Kansas Press, 1946, 151: Lawrence, Kansas.

malaria control. During the period where DDT was the main weapon used, PEP's purpose was to obtain an acceptance on the part of home owners and communities for its application at most several times a year. Today, the dominant technologies require individuals to change their daily behaviour, whether this is in terms of using bednets or seeking early treatment. In this context, PEP is a necessity and, because of this, there is greater attention being given to assessing the knowledge that people have concerning malaria and in the development of educational approaches that aim to bring about desired changes. However, as discussed in this chapter, PEP is largely to be found in demonstration projects and research studies; it has yet to become part of the main stream either for malaria control or for any other aspect of health, thus its status in future control efforts is uncertain.

Italian PEP Experience

The 20th century began with a fine example of health education and community participation in malaria control. Before World War I (WWI), malaria control was part of the Italian government's broad approach to social welfare that included:

The establishment of rural health stations whose function of administering quinine required constant contact with the populace, providing opportunities for individual persuasion, group instruction, house visits, and inspection tours of workplaces. These stations were seen as "apostles of health and hygiene."[3]

The teaching of leaders of the malaria campaign that "malaria could be successfully defeated only if workers were educated, properly nourished, hygienically housed, guaranteed productive work, and well organized in defense of their rights."[4]

The distribution of leaflets and posters to explain the mechanisms of malaria and the proper role of quinine. Newspapers publishing articles on all facets of state quinine. Doctors conducting speaking tours in rural areas, and journals publishing lectures which explain basic malariology in simple language.[5]

The inclusion of malaria in the curriculum of peasant schools. In classes on geography, for example, there were numerous opportunities to point out the malarial zones of the nation and of the locality, to explain the seriousness of the problem, and to discuss the mechanisms of transmission and the ways people could protect themselves.[6] More generally, the curriculum included "instruction of

[3] F.M. Snowden *The Conquest of Malaria, Italy, 1900–1962*, Yale University Press, 2006, 59: New Haven.
[4] Snowden, *The Conquest of Malaria, Italy, 1900–1962, op. cit.*, 63.
[5] Snowden, *The Conquest of Malaria, Italy, 1900–1962, op. cit.*, 75.
[6] Snowden, *The Conquest of Malaria, Italy, 1900–1962, op. cit.*, 79.

a kind that will enlighten our young people with regard to the etiology and pathogenesis of malaria, on the economic consequences that it produces, and on the means that exist to protect oneself from it."[7]

In the aftermath of WWI, the fascists in Italy came to power and developed a totally different approach to malaria control, one in which the people's 'education' and 'participation' became instruments to promote fascist propaganda and to squelch political opposition.

Early Rockefeller Foundation Enthusiasm Concerning Popular Education

Upon its establishment in 1913, the Rockefeller Foundation opted to focus on "the advancement of public health through medical research and education, including the demonstration of known methods of treating and preventing disease."[8] The Rockefeller Sanitary Commission, organized in 1909 for the eradication of hookworm in America's South, changed its name to the International Sanitary Commission. Its program was to extend to other countries and people "the work of eradicating hookworm disease as opportunity offers." Wickliffe Rose, an educator who had been in charge of the earlier sanitary commission, took over as director of the international commission. Rose, in his annual report for 1915, indicated that the significance of these early efforts "was not to be found in any expectation that the organization and funds at its disposal can complete the task of controlling or eradicating the formidable disease ..., but rather in certain characteristic policies to which the success of attending the previous work of the Commission may be attributed:"[9]

The need to work through governmental agencies and in cooperation with the medical profession, i.e. "through those agencies which the people regard as their own and on which the ultimate responsibility must inevitably rest."

Reliance upon popular education and on stimulating the interest of the common people rather than upon official exhortation or legislation to enforce measures essential to the public health.

Demonstrating in a limited area the feasibility of bringing disease under complete control.

Laying constant emphasis on the necessity of keeping the cost of the work down to a point so low that the feasibility of maintaining the work out of the

---

[7] *Ibid.*
[8] The Rockefeller Foundation, *Annual Report 1913–1914*, 11.
[9] The Rockefeller Foundation, *Annual Report 1915*, 14.

available public and private resources will become ultimately high, even if not at first apparent.

Rose was a strong advocate of popular education. He believed that it was possible to educate the people "however illiterate they may be, and to secure their interested cooperation in public health measures... An illiterate peasantry may, after all, be pretty intelligent... Getting officialdom in line," on the other hand, he regarded it as being "vastly more difficult."[10] Rose was sensitive to how people learned, as exemplified by his description of how, during the hookworm campaign, people "lingered and gathered in groups around a table of exhibits, exchanged experiences, listened to stories of improvement of a person who had been treated, and returned home to tell their neighbors what they had seen or heard."[11]

WS Leathers, at a memorial service honoring Rose, portrayed Rose as "a great believer in teaching the people by demonstration." He used the public health system as a means of "educating the people through the children." Looking beyond hookworm, he thought that "if the people could be educated about their situation and responsibility with regard to this disease, they would be in a receptive mood for information about other preventable diseases."[12]

Not surprisingly, during the years that Rose was Director of what is now the International Health Board (IHB) of the Rockefeller Foundation, popular education featured prominently in the annual reports of the Foundation.[13] For example, that of 1915 which dedicated two pages to a description of the hookworm disease exhibit prepared in San Francisco that lasted for nine months, before becoming a permanent exhibit at the Army Medical Museum in Washington. In the 1916 report, "satisfactory printed matter and exhibit material for use of field officers" were described as being "increasingly urgent."[14]

The tuberculosis control program in France, which began in 1917, provided another example of the importance given to public education on the part of the Foundation. A most impressive educational campaign was mounted which involved all kinds of approaches, but with particular emphasis given to reaching out to children. Two pages of the 1919 report were given to a description of how traditional Punch and Judy shows were used to reach 67,000 French children.

---

[10] Rose to Gunn, 17 January 1921, RAC, RF, Record Group 1.1, Series 712, Box 1, Folder 3.

[11] Quote from Link W, *The Paradox of Southern Progressivism*, The University of North Carolina Press, 1992, 148: Chapel Hill.

[12] Hackett's notes, RAC, RF, Record Group 3, Series 908, Box 3, 67.

[13] The International Health Commission was renamed the IHB in 1916. In 1927, it became the International Health Division.

[14] The Rockefeller Foundation, *Annual Report 1916*, 57.

Although popular education also featured in some malaria control programs present in the American South, the Foundation's Annual Reports did not highlight these activities.[15]

IHB's New Orientation Under New Leadership

Rose left the IHB in 1923; he was succeeded by Frederick F. Russell, who Rose had recruited in 1919 to develop a laboratory service in the countries where the IHD was working. Had the early disease control efforts, which featured health education, been a resounding success, Russell might have been forced to keep popular education and participation in the forefront of the IHD's program. But this was not the case.

Although Lewis Hackett later judged that hookworm was the "best" disease that Rose could have chosen as an entering wedge for a long-term public health program, being superior to both malaria and yellow fever for there were "no mysteries about the nature of the hookworm or the way it spread," it proved harder to control than anticipated.[16] By 1924, in fact, the RF concluded that there was a "lack of scientific information on certain points concerning which definite knowledge is indispensable if complete control is to be achieved."[17] Russell maintained that "defective scientific information" had led to the belief that hookworm could be "cleaned up in a short time."[18]

The sentiment that hookworm was inadequately understood before undertaking efforts to "change the habits in our South," was perhaps the reason why "Rose selected Russell" as his successor; the "lack of investigation" attributed to the time when Rose was in charge, "was a defect of the organization."[19] This was Hackett's conclusion. Hackett also judged that in 1913, there was "all too scanty knowledge of the epidemiology of the diseases to be attacked ... (and) the drugs and tools and other measures available proved very ineffective to control, not to speak of eradicating any of them."[20]

---

[15] See, for example, M. Humphreys *Malaria: Poverty, Race and Public Health in the United States*, The Johns Hopkins University Press, 2001, 131–9: Baltimore.

[16] L.W. Hackett, Once upon the time, presidential address, *American Journal of Tropical Medicine and Hygiene*, **9**, 107.

[17] The Rockefeller Foundation, *Annual Report 1924*, 157.

[18] Staff Conference notes, 13 January 1930, RAC, RF, Record Group 3, Series 908, Box 12, Folder 125, 2.

[19] Hackett's notes, RAC, RF, Record Group 3, Series 908, Box 3, 12.

[20] Hackett, Once upon the time, presidential address, *American Journal of Tropical Medicine and Hygiene*, **9**, 106.

Giving prominence to health education was pushed aside, yielding its importance to the need to increase technical knowledge concerning diseases and to improve upon the available control measures. What did remain a constant was the stress laid by the Foundation upon their broad policy of "demonstrating the practicability of controlling certain diseases... by fostering the development of governmental health agencies."[21]

So dramatic had Fred Russell's impact been on the work of the IHD that by the end of the decade he reported, with no explanation, that *nothing* had been done in "educating the public."[22] According to Russell, the IHD policy was "never" to attempt to "cover the whole field of public health," having limited its activities to those in which it possessed "special knowledge," or which promised "worthwhile results."[23] Furthermore, governments were never encouraged to set up an organization "limited as to subject"; instead, they should be "especially able in one field but should be competent to carry out a general program." By denying that the IHD possessed special knowledge concerning the whole field of public health, he provided a convenient justification for the lack of RF interest in this field of PEP. The Foundation did have such knowledge, but that is another story, not to be discussed further in this chapter.[24]

Neglect of Italian Experience by Foundation's Malarialogists

Neither Lewis Hackett nor Paul Russell, both very prominent Foundation malarialogists, acknowledged the early Italian experience in their historical accounts concerning malaria. Hackett reduced the Italian experience to one of distributing quinine; a time-honored resource, with a "history of three hundred years of constant defeat."[25] Russell, in his book *Man's Mastery of Malaria,* summarized Italy's efforts in one sentence: "by 1910, after very determined attempts to use this method of drug prophylaxis, it had to be admitted that it was not without serious defects."[26]

When Hackett arrived in Italy in 1924, there was nothing for him to see of pre-WWI PEP-related activities. In any case, his concern was with demonstrating the possibility of controlling malaria by controlling the *anopheles* vectors that

---

[21] May 1925 RF Board Meeting, RAC, RF, Record Group 3, Series 908, Box 12, Folder 128, 42.

[22] Staff Conference, 8 October 1930 , RAC, RF, Record Group 3, Series 908, Box 12, Folder 125.

[23] Outline IHD Presentation, October 1930, RAC, RF, Record Group 3, Series 908, Box 11, Folder 123.

[24] See, for example, Socrates Litsios, *Selskar 'Mike' Gunn and Public Health Reform in Europe, Of Medicine and Men. Biographies and Ideas in Social Hygiene in Europe between the War*, Peter Lang publisher, 2008: Frankfort.

[25] L.Hackett, *Malaria in Europe*, Oxford University Press, 1937, 20: London.

[26] P. Russell, *Man's Mastery of Malaria*, Oxford University Press, 1955, 135: London.

carried the disease. Very quickly he found himself at odds with malariologists from the League of Nations who were skeptical of the value of mosquito control and who, instead, favored tackling malaria as part of wider social uplift efforts, as Italy had done earlier in the century. At the time, this represented the 'modern view' of malariologists, whose leader was the Englishman S. Price James.

According to James, malaria, like tuberculosis and syphilis, was a "social disease."[27] As such, it should not be dealt with "as an isolated problem separate from either social, medical and public health affairs, or without the aid of educational arrangements designed to get the people to understand, and be willing to take advantage of, medical and sanitary measures established for their benefit."[28] He cited, as an example of 'social' means, England's history of introducing quinine into general practice and its "progressive cheapening until it could be bought directly from chemists by the poorer classes..."[29]

Hackett, in his influential book *Malaria in Europe,* labelled any resort to "general measures of social uplift and hygienic betterment" as tantamount "to a confession of ignorance or defeat."[30] His approach to the malaria problem left no room for any importance to be given to improving people's knowledge concerning malaria. Nor did he even assign any responsibility to the health officer to assess what the population knew or thought it knew concerning malaria. Hackett's description of how a health officer should go about appraising a malaria situation was largely a description of the technical difficulties in assessing the importance of the infection in a population. Revealingly, he referred to "social conditions" as constituting a "much vaguer field of inquiry."[31] Earlier in his career, Hackett indicated that he believed in "education," but "with backward people," the application of a "strict enforcement of a sanitary code, whether the people thoroughly understand it or not," was called for, adding further, "this is easier in a colony or under a mandate than in a democracy."[32]

For Hackett, the most important question of all was: "What is the economic condition of the population, how is it housed and fed, is it poor, crowded, or overworked." In seeking to answer this question, however, he indicated that "we are no

---

[27] S.P. James, The disappearance of malaria from England, *Proceedings of the Royal Society of Medicine,* 25 October 1929, 85.

[28] *Ibid.*

[29] *Ibid*, 82.

[30] Hackett, *Malaria in Europe, op.cit.,* 268.

[31] Hackett, *Malaria in Europe, op.cit.,* 261.

[32] Hackett to Gunn, 25 March, 1925, cited in P. Zylbmerman, A Transatlantic Dispute — The Etiology of Malaria and the Redesign of the Mediterranean Landscape, in *Shifting Boundaries of Public Health — Europe in the Twentieth Century* (Edited by Susan Gross Solomon, Lion Murard, and Patrick Zylberman), University of Rochester Press, 2008.

longer on solid ground. We have cut loose from our experimental data and become engaged at once in a battle of opinion...."[33] Hackett's facts were those of ecology of the mosquito; he used his facts to support his conclusion that malaria is "an entomological rather than a social problem."[34] Both he and Paul Russell, as indicated above, showed no interest in gathering facts in support of the thesis that malaria is also a social disease.

While Hackett had to contend with those who believed that malaria was part of a wider problem of inequity and had to be addressed as such, the views of Paul Russell, who was 10 years younger than Hackett, were shaped by a different history.

By contrast, Russell's view was that "without sufficient health-knowledge among laymen, personal and community hygiene is impossible."[35] This was consistent with the project that Russell initiated in the early 1930s in the Philippines, where, feeling "strongly that control work must be locally desired and locally carried out," he wished to engage community leaders in the development of local control schemes.[36] Although this project lasted for no more than one or two years, it did lead Russell to develop *A Malaria Primer* to be used by students and teachers. This primer was in "the nature of a profusely illustrated elementary handbook."[37]

Wickliffe Anderson's research on the Philippines led him to conclude that Russell's experience there led him to turn "away from the frustrations of 'race development' and concentrate(d) on manipulating the nonhuman elements of disease ecology, on fighting mosquitoes."[38] My own interpretation of his moving away from community involvement to technical aspects of malaria control was his frustration with the lack of interest on the part of public health officials in getting their hands dirty in the field. Without the interest and involvement of local public health officials, there was little chance of moving forward with any kind of participatory strategy. Revealingly, within a year, he identified "an automatic or biological weapon" as "an outstanding need in the Tropics today."[39]

---

[33] Hackett, *Malaria in Europe, op.cit.*, 261.

[34] Hackett, *Malaria in Europe, op.cit.*, 10.7.

[35] P.F. Russell, Some social obstacles to malaria control, *Indian Medical Gazette*, November 1941, 681–90.

[36] Cited in Wickliffe Anderson, *Colonial Pathologies: American Tropical Medicine, Race, and Hygiene in the Philippines*, Duke University Press, 2006, 221: Durham.

[37] The Rockefeller Foundation, *Annual Report 1932*, 79. Unfortunately, I have not been able to locate a copy of this publication nor even the short articles that Russell wrote in which he described it.

[38] Anderson, *Colonial Pathologies, op.cit.*, 233. "Race development" is the language of Anderson, not that of Russell.

[39] P.F. Russell, *Malaria in the Philippine Islands*, 176.

Russell left the Philippines in 1934 and went to Madras, India where he concentrated his attention on searching for such a weapon. Effective and affordable weapons were unavailable when he chaired the 1937 Bandoeng Conference's technical committee on malaria. The lack of successful projects was cited as the reason for "official apathy and failure to appropriate funds for control programmes." Thus, the need for "practical demonstrations of malaria control as a means of arousing interest of lay (and even health) administrations."[40] The committee envisaged a role for the "people themselves" in "minor control methods."[41]

In his preface to Marshall Barber's autobiography, Russell acknowledged Barber's half-century effort in chasing malaria plasmodia and their *anopheles* in "more countries than any other malariologist of record," and Barber's role in discovering the anti-larval effects of Paris Green and for improving the precipitin test.[42] Russell chose to ignore Barber's call for popular education, even though it was the main message in Barber's conclusion, in which he outlined how he would teach children health through "natural history."[43] He would use simple means, for example, by setting a fruit-jar in the schoolroom window, "where pupils could see the various stages of mosquito development — elementary instruction which would prepare their minds for learning the rudiments of malaria transmission."[44]

Post-WWII Developments

With the arrival of DDT the prospects for malaria control changed dramatically. Almost overnight, eradication became a goal that appeared to some to be feasible. But the early success with DDT raised a new problem, one not encountered by any health program previously, namely an explosive population growth following the success of malaria control efforts using DDT, as witnessed in Ceylon in the 1940s. This led many to question the priority being given to malaria control.[45] Russell studied very carefully the extensive literature that surround this subject, as well as

---

[40] League of Nations, *Report of the Intergovernmental Conference* on Far-*Eastern Countries on Rural Hygiene*, League of Nations, 1937, 90: Geneva.

[41] *Ibid*, 92.

[42] Barber, *op.cit.*, 7.

[43] Barber, *op. cit.*, 152.

[44] *Ibid*. Other examples of educating children about malaria include efforts in Zululand where schools included a weekly nature study on mosquitoes in the 1930s and earlier efforts in Indonesia where children were taught to recognize different mosquito species (see Litsios, S. *The Tomorrow of Malaria*, New Zealand Pacific Press, 1996: Wellington).

[45] See Litsios S, Malaria control, the Cold War, and the postwar reorganization of international assistance, *Medical Anthropology*, 1997, **17**(3): 255–78.

other books that looked at the human condition from a more holistic viewpoint. In a matter of days in the early 1950s he read, and commented on:

J.D. Bernal — The Social Function of Science

Josué de Castro — *Geography of Hunger* (comment: interesting but marred by bad logic, false biology, historical dishonesty, self-righteousness, and even malice ... like Russell, Vogt, Osborne and "many so many others today, has 'a touch of hysteria in his blood'.")[46]

A.G. Mezerik — *The Pursuit of Plenty* (*comment*: gives some of the facts of life without playing on the theme of fear)[47]

Fairfield Osborne — *Our Plundered Planet*

Bertrand Russell — *New Hopes for a Changing World* (*comment*: worth reading)[48]

René Sand — *Health and Human Progress* (*comment*: must be a classic)[49]

William Vogt — *Road to Survival* (*comment*: amazingly good and amazingly bad — his terms 'the dangerous doctor' and 'ecologically ignorant sanitarians' suggest that he himself is a 'sociologically ignorant biologist.' He fails to realize the weight of organization of the population.)[50]

Norbert Weiner — *The Human Use of Human Beings* (*comment*: an irritating book that seemed to be working up to an important climax but then faded away)[51]

Russell concluded: "That physicians, malariologists, and sanitarians integrate their activities with those of agriculturists, demographers, social scientists, economists, educators, political and religious leaders is of the utmost importance. For only thus can there be joint planning of social reorientation that will result not in bigger populations but in healthier communities. In this way, there will be accelerated progress towards higher planes of health and living."[52]

PEP did not feature prominently in the guidance provided by the WHO malaria expert committee concerning eradication. This did not mean that it did not feature in national programs, but as an eradication campaign was a highly centralized, military-like operation, the aim of PEP was to get the people to accept the campaign, not

[46] P. Russell diary entry 4 March 1952.
[47] P. Russell diary entry 26 February 1952.
[48] P. Russell diary entry 1 March 1952.
[49] P. Russell diary entry 27 February 1952.
[50] P. Russell diary entry 26 February 1952.
[51] P. Russell diary entry 28 February 1952.
[52] P. Russell, *Man's Mastery of Malaria*, op.cit., 257.

to participate actively in its activities. Looking back on this period, one senior WHO malariologist judged the impact of health education for malaria control to be "minimal" for a variety of reasons, including the fact that it had not been properly conducted, as it did not pay "adequate attention ... to learning processes for the populations concerned."[53]

PEP in the post-Eradication period (1970–1990)

An interregional conference held in Brazzaville in 1972, which addressed the question on how to control malaria where "time-limited eradication" was judged to be "impracticable at present," is notable for the attention given to health education, and the recognition given to the "great potential" that exists in rural communities for "self-help in improving their health conditions when well motivated and approached through proper health education."[54] The report included considerable detail concerning educational approaches used in Ethiopia, and proposed, as suitable community-level activities, drug distribution to particularly vulnerable groups, improvement of housing conditions, and the carrying out of minor source-reduction operations. Most importantly, the conference recommended that "pilot studies be promoted on motivating rural communities to undertake self-help activities on malaria control."[55]

The 16th Malaria Expert Committee, that met a year later, did not follow-up on the call for self-help pilot studies. Health education was "essential"[56], but its responsibility rested "with the basic health services."[57] However, none of the functions identified by the Committee as important for the health services addressed popular education or participation. The local level, being closest to the community, instead of leading PEP efforts, were assigned the job of gathering data for the higher levels, applying control measures, maintaining equipment and "maintaining discipline and submitting proposals concerning rewards and disciplinary measures."[58] A military-like approach to control, it would seem, was still the dominating mentality. In such a context, it is not surprising that PEP received little if no attention.

---

[53] G. Gramiccia, Health education in malaria control — why has it failed?, *World Health Forum*, 1981, **2**(3), 385–93.

[54] Malaria Control in Countries where Time-Limited Eradication is Impracticable at Present, *Report of a WHO Interregional Conference (WHO Technical Report Series, No. 537)*, World Health Organization, 1974, 53: Geneva.

[55] *Ibid*, 53.

[56] *Ibid*, 16.

[57] *Ibid*, 19.

[58] WHO Expert Committee on Malaria, *Sixteenth Report (WHO Technical Report Series, No. 549)*, World Health Organization, 1974, 43: Geneva.

However, in the same report, but under the subject of "the cost of malaria control programmes," there is a brief discussion of the potential for enlisting "those networks of voluntary, community, and public participation that exist outside the official government-sponsored health service."[59] Malaria programmes had "extensive experience" in the development of "voluntary village collaboration," but no references were provided. Revealingly, it was acknowledged that malaria planners had not yet begun "to explore, on a large scale, the cooperative potential of non-formal traditional indigenous health service system, including the indigenous midwife, the traditional rural practitioner, and other forms of traditional community social organization."[60]

These latter excerpts illustrate a phenomenon often found in such reports, namely, the presence of different voices, some neutral at best to the role of the community, others enthusiastic. This is somewhat reminiscent of the Bandoeng report where Paul Russell wrote the report of the malaria committee, while Selskar Gunn wrote the overall summary, where he addressed malaria control in the language of social medicine.[61]

The same ambiguity was present during the discussions held by 17th session of the Expert Committee (1979) concerning the implication of the newly adopted policy of primary health care for malaria control. One senior WHO official discussed community participation strictly in terms of intersectoral coordination, thus indicating very clearly a top-heavy orientation to the subject. The head of the India program admitted that community participation had never been tried in India, even though it was recommended in a policy from 1947. Bruce-Chwatt, glossed over the whole subject by indicating to Dr. Halfdan Mahler (WHO Director-General) that he (Mahler) was "speaking to the converted."[62] As it was, none of the attention given to the subject when Mahler was present appeared in the final report. There, the recommendation concerning the "role and place of malaria services, general health services, and the community," was for WHO to "evaluate the experiences gained in various countries on the integration of malaria control within basic health services and make this information available to Member countries."[63] Behind this recommendation was the belief shared by most malariologists, despite

---

[59] *Ibid*, 28.

[60] *Ibid*.

[61] See S. Litsios, Selskar Gunn and Paul Russell of the Rockefeller Foundation: A Contrast in Styles and Malaria and International Health Organizations in Benjamin B Page and David A Valone (editors) *Philanthropic Foundations and the Globalization of Scientific Medicine and Public Health*, University Press of America: Lanham, Maryland.

[62] Personal notes.

[63] WHO Expert Committee on Malaria, *Seventeenth Report (WHO Technical Report Series, No. 640)*, World Health Organization, 1979, 61: Geneva.

Bruce-Chwatt's claim, that PHC offered no panacea for malaria control. No doubt this discussion confirmed what Mahler had concluded two years earlier, namely, that "it was probably a mistake to stipulate that 'global eradication' remained the objective when it was obviously out of reach for decades to come, with the means at our disposal."[64]

While the WHO expert committee seemed hesitant to pursue a pro-PEP agenda, USAID moved forcibly in that direction. In the spring of 1975 a mission reviewed African malaria, seeking to determine vector control methods that might be used at the local level, with particular attention given to actions which could be conducted on a "community or self-help basis rather than with the rigid central direction required for a malaria eradication campaign."[65] WHO malariologists visits on the way to Africa evoked a "general attitude of scepticism that self-help schemes at the village level could work." On the other hand, US specialists in primary health care were much more up-beat concerning self-help, and emphasized the importance of locals being responsible for whatever actions organized.

Their visit to Kenya and Nigeria (one month in total), led them to conclude that "any malaria control would have to be carried out as a part of the(se) health services ... It appears that the people would reject a program designed only for the control of malaria." They recommended that AID support "a small scale research project to determine the effectiveness of a combination of self-help methods for control of malaria." Such a project should explore screening (where practical), bednets, distribution of pyrethrum sprays and coils, and the dispensing of antimalarial drugs." Kenya seemed a suitable site for such a demonstration project.[66]

USAID went on to develop a manual on malaria control in primary health care in Africa. Contrary to the earlier emphasis on vector control, this manual gave highest priority to "maximum extension of cost-efficient mortality reduction through chemotherapy."[67] The section devoted to health education and community participation noted that the use of educational methods to change individual and community beliefs and behavior was "basic to PHC." The purposes of educational activities may be to stimulate appreciation of early treatment, motivate compliance with chemotherapeutic regimens, and, when appropriate, motivate villagers to adopt new patterns of behaviour that might reduce the likelihood of infections at a later time. In the final analysis, however, "the ultimate success of the program

---

[64] *Development of the antimalaria programme: report by the Ad Hoc Committee on Malaria of the Executive Board (EB57/19, Annex 2)*, World Health Organization, 1976: Geneva.

[65] Report of Consultants — African Malaria Office of Health, (TA/H), AID, 1975.

[66] See, for example, the special issue of the *Annals of Tropical Medicine*, 1987, **81** (Suppl 1) devoted to the Saradidi project in rural Kenya.

[67] *Manual on Malaria Control in Primary Health Care in Africa*. Bureau for Africa, USAID, December, 1982: Washington, DC.

will depend less upon the message from outside the community than upon the extent to which community leaders and organizations are able to develop support for the program and understanding of its details on the part of the community residents."

An AID malaria strategy workshop, held in June 1983, explored further the implications of the PHC approach for malaria control.[68] It concluded that in endemic areas where malaria was a major threat to economic development or quality of life, AID "should provide selective support of malaria control using the most satisfactory available vehicle," which in many countries would be the PHC system. An AID strategy assisting malaria control through PHC should include a community participation component which would support "operational research into techniques for eliciting increased community participation in malaria control." AID support for national training of PHC and malaria workers in concepts and methods for developing and implementing educational approaches was deemed "appropriate." Such approaches should emphasize preventive and protective actions that individuals and communities could take for malaria control, such as the reduction of sources for vector breeding, physical personal protection techniques (screens, bednets, repellents), effective use of drugs and early notification to and contact with primary health workers and malaria workers for treatment.

Later in 1983, a WHO Study Group on Malaria Control as part of Primary Health Care considered the planning of malaria control in that context and, particularly, the collective experience of countries, in order to identify practical approaches that could be applied at various levels and those which needed to be further developed.[69] A study group differs from an Expert Committee in that its subject is somewhat problematic, requiring further study, which the group is expected to define. Despite the fact that all regions of the world were represented, some participants felt that the subject applied only to Africa.[70]

The group explored the same issues that USAID had been investigating, in particular the role of the community in antimalaria activities, which it saw as requiring the promotion of the general awareness of the community of the importance of prompt and effective treatment of malaria cases, for which community health workers needed to possess the necessary diagnostic skills and technical and supervisory support. Individuals in the community should be motivated to use

---

[68] *AID Malaria Strategy Workshop, June 7–10,* 1983, published by Insect Control & Research, INC., September 1983: Columbia, Maryland.

[69] Malaria control as part of primary health care, *Report of a WHO Study Group (WHO Technical Report Series, No. 712)*, World Health Organization, 1984: Geneva.

[70] Personal observation. I even overheard several members contemplating abandoning the meeting as a protest to this effect!

mosquito nets, repellents, etc., as safeguards against malaria. Countries were urged to support efforts to create community awareness and involvement in activities affecting the quality of life.

In September 1985, the WHO Expert Committee on Malaria considered approaches to implementing antimalaria action within developing primary health care systems. A somewhat different approach to the subject was adopted, one that looked at all technical and managerial aspects of malaria, including, e.g., the management of severe and complicated malaria. The central focus was on the health services, with little specific attention on the community as such. In his opening statement to the meeting, the responsible WHO Assistant Director-General indicated that the "training of health workers at all levels had to be considered not only in general terms with respect to epidemiology and control of malaria, but also in very specific terms, particularly at the field level, in relation to the duties to be carried out for malaria control by health workers. These workers should support communities that were attempting community malaria control as well as educating individuals and groups to participate in, and contribute actively to, the control efforts. Research and development studies would be needed to ascertain to what extent non-professional workers, guided and supervised by personnel at the first referral level, who, in turn, were advised by experts in malaria, could be trained to cope with these tasks in addition to their other activities."[71]

The committee's response to this was to include a recommendation concerning research and development, which, in addition to the study of approaches to training non-professional workers to cope with antimalaria activities on top of their other activities, included: factors influencing community participation and intersectoral cooperation; appropriate implementation at the community level of malaria control, control of other priority diseases, and other primary health care activities, including studies of whether (or where) such activities could be carried out by a multipurpose community health worker, or whether malaria control activities should be divided among a number of categories of worker, such as those dealing with disease control and those dealing with other promotional and preventive activities, i.e., those dealing with people and those dealing with the environment; and ways of developing and promoting the popular, habitual use of simple, safe, cheap, and effective methods to be used by individuals and communities for their own protection against disease vectors.

Aware of the fact that in many areas of Africa private channels of distribution of antimalarial drugs reached the periphery more effectively than did the health services, they recommended that the health service concentrate its efforts on

---

[71] Expert Committee on Malaria, *Eighteenth report (WHO Technical Report Series, No. 735)*, World Health Organization, 1986, 8: Geneva.

providing adequate information about the use of drugs, improving accessibility to appropriate treatment, and eventually regulating and controlling the drug trade.

This report, perhaps more than any other, clearly indicates the difficulties facing any malaria control policy that accepts the requirement of total integration with health services that are oriented towards the primary health care approach. First, and foremost, for a broad-based control strategy to evolve that is sensitive to the specific epidemiological situations faced by each malarious community there must be in place a hierarchical system which functions extraordinarily well, i.e., information from the periphery serving to fine-tune strategies adopted at the central level, but which allow for their implementation in a manner that is sensitive to the specifics of each locality, and, most importantly, used in such a fashion as to encourage community participation. The technical problems facing both treatment and vector control, e.g. growing resistance of the parasites to drugs and the mosquitoes to insecticides, made developing such a system far more difficult, which no doubt accounts for the fact that at the end of the meeting, its Chairman, Sir Ian McGregor, was heard remarking that what we have produced represents "an act of faith!"[72]

The next Expert Committee meeting (the 19th session), which took place in 1989, but whose report was never officially published,[73] while covering similar ground as the previous session, did explicitly explore the issue of public education and information. For what I believe may be the first time, the malaria expert committee made explicit the responsibility of malaria control managers regarding health education, namely that "those responsible for malaria control develop working relations with focal points responsible for health education at all levels of the health system."[74] Hitherto, one was left with the impression (rightly or wrongly) that the malariologists did not want to get involved with health education as such. The committee also stressed the point that communities could not solve the malaria problem on their own through self-protection and community prevention activities, as there is a need for timely diagnostic and therapeutic services, including a referral system capable of managing treatment failures and severe and complicated malaria cases, functions which only a well-established health system can provide.

The importance given to diagnostic services and treatment facilities led the committee to recommend that, since self-treatment is practiced in most

---

[72] Personal notes.

[73] Why this report was never published as part of WHO's TRS series is not clear, other than the fact that there were important differences of opinion within the WHO Secretariat concerning certain aspects.

[74] WHO Expert Committee on Malaria, *Nineteenth Report*, WHO document WHO/CTD/92.1, 43.

communities, "all possible channels should be used to teach the proper use of drugs, including community leaders, traditional birth attendants, pharmacists or drug vendors, school teachers and radio broadcasters, as well as health profession-als (including private practitioners)."[75] The committee did not address the educa-tion of family members, despite the fact American experience in Africa had led their malariologists to conclude that "parents and communities must be involved in the process of disease recognition, therapy, and prevention" if the existing pat-terns of childhood morbidity and mortality were to be improved.[76]

The issue of self-treatment was addressed in the late 1970s within the WHO by the health education program.[77] Its importance for malaria should have been picked up at that time, but it was not.[78] One possible reason for its omission is the strong sense among the senior WHO malariologists that mothers should not be considered as 'front-line' workers, an issue that arose during the 19th session and which divided the participants, as well as some of the secretariat.[79]

The modern era (1990–today)

In view of the continuing seriousness of the malaria situation, WHO's Executive Board in 1990 proposed that a Ministerial Conference on Malaria be held to encourage affected countries and the international community to intensify efforts to control the disease. After preparatory meetings involving representatives of donor agencies, research institutions, the United Nations and its specialized agen-cies, as well as managers, scientists and administrators, a consensus was reached on current standards for malaria control and a Global Malaria Control Strategy was formulated.[80] The strategy had little to say concerning PEP-related issues; communities were "to be full partners in malaria control activities" and "appropri-ate education" was advised for women's groups and among schoolchildren, as

---

[75] *Ibid*, 53.

[76] J.G. Breman and C.C. Campbell, Combating severe malaria in African children, *Bulletin of the World Health Organisation*, 1988, **66**(5) 611–20.

[77] See, for example, L.S. Leven, *Self-care: lay initiatives in health, based on the proceedings of a Symposium on the Role of the Individual in Primary Health Care*, organized by the Joint Center for Studies of Health Programs, Copenhagen, in collaboration with the Sandoz Institute and Socio-Economic Studies, 1979, 2nd ed.: Geneva.

[78] I share some responsibility in this omission. As the designated 'coordinator' between the PHC unit (where I was a programme area leader) and the malaria action programme, it was just as much my responsibility to raise the issue as it was that of the malaria programme.

[79] I frankly was shocked that my director was one of those who opposed this, contrary to the USAID position as pushed by the American member of the committee.

[80] *A global strategy for malaria control*, World Health Organization, 1993: Geneva.

education "enhances awareness and skills, empowering people to be active partners in malaria control." The Global Strategy was presented to and endorsed by
the Ministerial Conference on Malaria, which was held in Amsterdam, Netherlands,
in October 1992. Subsequently, it was endorsed by the UN and ECOSOC.

In 1998 WHO initiated the Roll Back Malaria project. The global malaria
action plan produced by the Roll Back Malaria (RBM) program gives prominence
to "communication and behaviour change methodologies."[81] Early on an excellent
publication (Community involvement in rolling back malaria)[82] described in some
detail the various roles that the community could play in malaria control, including
experiences to that effect. Interestingly, the key individuals involved were
Ethiopians with medical and social science backgrounds, with knowledge of the
experience of their country that had been recognized in the Brazzaville meeting
cited above. The RBM plan calls for "more dedicated funding for communication
activities" at the international, national and the community levels; especially in
light of the numerous "gaps" present in the current malaria communication
structure.[83]

The same year that the RBM program was launched, the 20th session of the
malaria expert committee met to review progress and make recommendations
concerning malaria control. The committee noted the success achieved through the
use of insecticide-treated materials, which, while not being new, had progressed
significantly during the 1990s. It reiterated the importance of decentralization
which included an empowerment of local authorities and communities to identify
their priorities and needs, adding that "health issues should be addressed directly
through enhanced community awareness and knowledge about disease prevention,
diagnosis and treatment as well as through local operational research activities."[84]
On the other hand, it noted that poorly managed decentralization of malaria
control programs had undermined their effectiveness and hampered their ability
to fulfill their responsibilities. Experienced staff had retired or moved to other
positions thus leaving programs poorly prepared to guide operations at the community level.

The committee noted that the costs of extending public health services to the
community level had accelerated the process of involvement by communities and
the private sector as partners in malaria control, and that this could be expected to

---

[81] The Global Malaria Action Plan for a malaria-free world. (http://www.rbm.who.int/gmap/),
210–5.
[82] *Community involvement in rolling back malaria*, WHO document WHO/CDS/RBM/2002.42,
2002.
[83] *Global strategy, op.cit.*, 211.
[84] WHO Expert Committee on Malaria, *Twentieth Report (WHO Technical Report Series, No. 892)*,
World Health Organization, 2000: Geneva.

be a slow but continuous process. Information was becoming available, largely from Africa, south of the Sahara, on the cost-effectiveness of three types of interventions undertaken at the community level: the provision of widely available curative treatment, usually by village volunteers; chemoprophylaxis for pregnant women; and the use of insecticide-treated materials. Information is needed from different epidemiological settings on the simultaneous use of such interventions.

While community-based interventions were judged to offer hope for the future, it was difficult at that time to draw conclusions about the types of interventions that could successfully be delivered using community involvement. In spite of evidence that early treatment of malaria in children lowered case-fatality rates, it had proved difficult to design community-based distribution mechanisms that demonstrated an impact on mortality. While it was clear that insecticide-treated materials for all and chemoprophylaxis for pregnant women would save lives and were cost-effective in research settings, it was not yet known whether they could be delivered at low cost in a practical programme setting. Simultaneous use of two or more of these interventions, which might be possible as community involvement increased, offered promise of a synergistic effect on severe morbidity and mortality. This conclusion, in effect, outlined the operational research priorities that have engaged scientists ever since.

For the time being, however, and not for the first or last time, the question of what kind of popular education might be needed in support of community involvement was not addressed, other than the indication that the "university curricula for health workers" needed to address "the practical needs of malaria control (e.g. aiming to increase their awareness of information, education and communication needs of the community and the patient, and the concept of the Integrated Management of Childhood Illnesses)."[85] The history concerning this aspect of medical education is a long and torturous one that has proven the most difficult to bring about, a difficulty that has never prevented this or other expert committees from pointing out the imperativeness of its being overcome.

Numerous studies have been conducted during the last decade concerning community perception and knowledge of malaria. The results are somewhat disquieting. For example, people's knowledge about signs and symptoms of malaria was found "to be very poor" in one study carried out in Nigeria;[86] very few people in Nepal were

---

[85] Integrated management of childhood illness (IMCI) was launched by the World Health Organization and UNICEF in 1996 in recognition of the drawbacks and inefficiencies of the vertical non-integrated programme approach to child health.

[86] I.G. Ukpong, K.N. Opara, L.P.E. Usip and F.S. Ekpu, Community perceptions about malaria, mosquito and insecticide treated nets in rural community of the Niger Delta Nigeria: implications for control, *Research Journal of Parasitology*, 2007, **2**(1) 13–22.

aware that the treatment of malaria in time could save a life;[87] and 30% of respondents in one study in Kenya did not know that malaria was carried by mosquitoes and nearly 70% had poor knowledge of the habitat characteristics of malaria vectors.[88]

On the other hand, there have been new initiatives concerning PEP that are encouraging, e.g. the World Bank considering the incorporation of malaria control into school health, as part of an aim of promoting "health practices in the broader community and the use of school buildings themselves to improve access to appropriate prevention and treatment;"[89] improved knowledge of mosquito ecology and disease epidemiology, changes in agricultural practices, and an increase in environmentally sound measures for mosquito control and disease prevention following a 20-week pilot education program;[90] and the use of a 'malaria fact card' that improved treatment knowledge and prevention strategies in Tanzania.[91] Another positive development is the increased number of efforts being made to improve the quality of services provided by drug shops in sub-Saharan Africa. One study reviewed ten such educational efforts, but while evidence of improved knowledge was found, it was also learned that profit incentives appeared to influence (negatively) the level of success of educational interventions.[92]

Still, much of the literature describing current malaria control projects is void of any reference to PEP, thus leaving this author somewhat doubtful concerning the extent to which it is being used. Nevertheless, and of great importance, is the fact that the 'new' interventions of long-lasting insecticidal-treated nets (LLINs) and artemisinin-based combination therapies (ACTs) are having an impact on malaria incidence, which in some instances is quite dramatic.[93]

---

[87] A.B. Joshi and M.R. Banjara, Malaria-related knowledge, practices and behaviour of people in Nepal, *Journal of vector borne diseases*, March 2008, **45**(1) 44–50.

[88] S.S. Imbahale, U. Fillinger, A. Githeko, W.R. Mukabana and W. Takken, An exploratory survey of malaria prevalence and people's knowledge, attitudes and practices of mosquito larval source management for malaria control in western Kenya, *Acta Tropica*, September 2010, **115**(3), 248–56.

[89] INCORPORATING MALARIA CONTROL INTO SCHOOL HEALTH, Draft prepared for discussions by the World Bank, March 2003.

[90] J. Yasuoka, T.W. Mangione, A. Spielman and R. Levins, Impact of education on Knowledge, agricultural practices, and community action for mosquito control, and mosquito-borne disease prevention in rice ecosystems in Sri Lanka, *American Journal of Tropical Medicine and Hygiene*, 2006, **74**(6), 1034–42.

[91] M. Chambuso, V. Mugoyela and W. Kalala, Consumer survey of malaria fact card: an educational and communication tool in Tanzania, *East African journal of public health*, October 2007, **4**(2) 59–63.

[92] F.N. Wafula and C.A. Goodman, Are Interventions for improving the quality of services provided by specialized drug shops effective in sub-Africa? A systematic review of the literature, *International Journal for Quality in Health Care*, 2010, **22**(4) 316–23.

[93] E. Chizema-Kawesha, J.M. Miller, R.W. Steketee, V.M. Mukonka, C. Mukuka, D. Abdirahman, S.K. Miti and C.C. Cambell, Scaling up malara control in Zambia: progress and impact 2005–2008, *American Journal of Tropical Medicine and Hygiene*, 2010, **83**(3) 480–8.

Despite progress, however, there remain doubts in the minds of some concerning whether or not these developments are sustainable. Some of the literature concerning LLINs and ACTs reads like the 1950s literature concerning DDT, i.e. the hope for a magic-bullet hangs heavy in the air, but whether this implies that the "pendulum has swung decidedly toward narrower biomedical approaches aimed at eliminating the immediate causes of disease," or not, is not yet clear.[94]

Concluding Comments

History seems to suggest that PEP works best when carried out by dedicated individuals and organizations that are working in and with communities. But when one reads that "national leadership and ownership of community partnerships are essential ..." there is reason to believe that policy makers may still be enamored of top-down approaches that so much characterized the campaigns of the past.[95] Also, there remains a tendency to blame failures in the past on policies that favored a health agenda "structured around diseases and interventions rather than around the broader challenges being face by health systems."[96] The claim is that these policies have resulted in "fragmentation of the governance of the health sector."[97] Malaria program managers may find themselves, as they have in the past, facing the dilemma that the pursuit of 'their' interventions will be seen by other program managers as promoting fragmentation.

Marshall Barber's proposition that malaria could be controlled in one or two generations if suitable educational efforts were carried out has never been given a chance to be verified. Nor is it likely that such an experiment would be carried out in the current situation, especially as malaria control successes are being reported more frequently. Whether PEP will again be allowed to fall into oblivion, however, given these successes, is not clear. Hopefully, funding agencies and educational programs for health workers, beginning with medical doctors, will recognize the importance of PEP and incorporate it into their policies. Also, by necessity, PEP for malaria must be integrated with other PEP initiatives, thus serving to better integrate malaria with other health service priorities. Finally, investing in PEP can serve as a building block for future control activities, this is especially important if the ones in place today do not yield the results currently expected of them.

---

[94] R.M. Packard, *The Making of a Tropical Disease: A Short History of Malaria*, The Johns Hopkins University Press, 2007, 248: Baltimore.
[95] The UNICEF 2008 State of the Child Report, 44.
[96] World Health Report, 2008, 83.
[97] *Ibid.*

Part II

Scientific, Medical, and Public Health Perspectives

6 The Contribution of The Gambia to Malaria Research

Brian Greenwood

The Gambia, a small country on the West Coast of Africa, has played a more important role in research on malaria than might have been anticipated for a country of its size. This chapter describes some of the ways in which research conducted in The Gambia has contributed to knowledge of the biology of malaria infection and on how it can be controlled.

The Gambia

The Gambia, situated approximately 13^0 north of the equator, is the smallest country on mainland Africa with artificial borders defined during the colonial period (Figure 1). During the first half of the second millennium, the area now known as The Gambia was part of the large West African Kingdom of Mali. Portuguese explorers first reached the River Gambia in 1455 and established trading and missionary outposts around the mouth of the river but these were not sustained.[1] In 1588, exclusive trading rights were granted to English merchants by the Portuguese crown and in 1618, King James I[st] of England granted a charter to English merchants for trade with The Gambia, establishing the long association between the United Kingdom and The Gambia. During the seventeenth and eighteenth centuries, there were repeated outbreaks of hostilities between France and England over the territories around the Senegal and Gambia rivers which were not resolved until 1783 when the Treaty of Versailles ceded the Gambia River to Great Britain, leaving the French with a small enclave at Albreda which was finally ceded to Great Britain in 1856. During the nineteenth century, Great Britain

---

[1] J.M. Gray, *A History of the Gambia*, Frank Cass & Co., 1966: London.

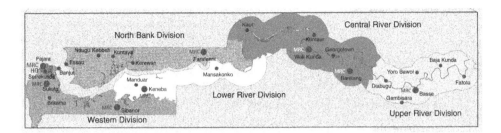

Figure 1. Map of The Gambia showing some of the sites mentioned in this chapter.

gradually extended its control over the area surrounding the river, establishing the capital, Bathurst (now Banjul) at its mouth in 1816, and a base on McCarthy Island approximately 150 miles upriver in 1823. Following the abolition of slavery throughout the British Empire in 1833, The Gambia was used as a base for interrupting the Atlantic slave trade and liberated slaves were resettled on McCarthy Island and at other centres in the country. The boundaries of The Gambia, which cut across the homelands of several ethnic groups, were finally delineated in 1889. The Gambia gained independence from the United Kingdom in 1965.

The Gambia covers an area of approximately 4,000 square miles and extends inwards from the Atlantic coast on either side of the River Gambia for about 250 miles (Figure 1). The climate of The Gambia is typical of the West African savannah with a short rainy season that lasts from June to October and a longer dry season. Rainfall averages around 800 mm a year and has fallen significantly during the past 100 years.[2] The population of The Gambia is about 1.7 million and is still predominantly rural, although the peri-urban population around the capital Banjul is expanding rapidly. The population belongs primarily to Mandinka, Wollof, Fula, Jollof or Serahule ethnic groups. Jollofs are probably the earliest residents of the central part of The Gambia with later immigrations of Mandinkas and Fulas from the east. Wollofs are concentrated on the coast. Maize, millet and rice are cultivated and cattle tolerant to trypanosomiasis make a valuable contribution to the economy. In recent years, tourism has become an important source of income, especially in the areas on the coast. The per capita GDP is approximately $500. Health services are provided through four government run hospitals, a system of dispensaries and a number of private clinics.

Nearly all malaria transmission in The Gambia occurs during the rainy season and the period immediately afterwards. *Plasmodium falciparum* is the dominant malaria parasite although *P. malariae* and *P. ovale* are also seen. *P. vivax* is not

---

[2]P. Hutchinson, Rainfall analysis of the Sahelian drought in the Gambia, *Journal of Climatology*, 1985, **5**, 665–72.

prevalent because a large majority of the indigenous population lack the red cell Duffy antigen necessary for invasion of red blood cells by this parasite. *Anopheles gambiae sl.* is the main mosquito vector.

Malaria in The Gambia in the Pre-colonial Period

Little is known about the early history of The Gambia but it is likely that the areas alongside the river have been settled for at least 2,000 years. The construction of elaborate stone circles on the north bank of the river Gambia (Figure 2) and in adjacent areas of Senegal around 600–800 AD suggests that there were well established agricultural communities in The Gambia at that time. The presence of settled communities, *anopheline* mosquitoes and a permissive climate make it almost certain that *falciparum* malaria was an important cause of mortality and morbidity in The Gambia in the pre-colonial period. A prevalence of sickle cell trait of around 15–20% in Gambians[3] suggests that malaria has exerted strong selection pressure on the population of The Gambia for many generations.

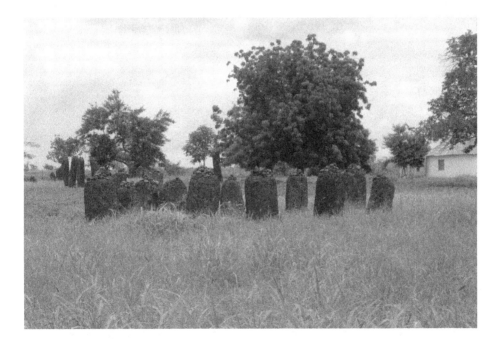

Figure 2.   A stone circle at Wassu, The Gambia, one of the many stone circles found in The Gambia and Senegal which are believed to have been set up around 750 AD. Their purpose is unknown.

[3]S. Bennett, E.M. Riley, P.A. Rowe, P.H. Jakobsen, A. O'Donnell, and B.M. Greenwood, Morbidity from malaria and immune responses to defined *Plasmodium falciparum* antigens in children with sickle cell trait in the Gambia, *Transactions of the Royal Society of Tropical Medicine and Hygiene*, 1992, **86**, 494–8.

Malaria in Colonial Times

The unhealthy nature of The Gambia was well recognised by early European traders who visited The Gambia to trade, first in commodities such as gold and beeswax and then in slaves. In an attempt to mitigate some of the risks to health posed by the climate, traders from Courland (Latvia) established a base on a small island in the centre of the river, called St Andrew's Island, in 1651. The island was renamed James Island when it was taken over by the British ten years later. A small fort was established on the island (Figure 3) which played an important role in the history of The Gambia during the following 150 years, changing hands on several occasions between pirates, the French and English.[4] Life expectation for those garrisoned on the island was extremely poor and there are many accounts of the poor health of those who survived, with fever (almost certainly malaria) and flux (dysentery) being the most important causes of severe illness and death.

In the eighteenth century, other trading bases were established further up river. One of these settlements, Pisania (Figure 4), was the base from which the explorer Mungo Park set out on two expeditions to find the source of the Nile, 'discovering' the Niger instead. Mungo Park was a surgeon and his diaries, which survived his death on the Niger, provide an account of many of the

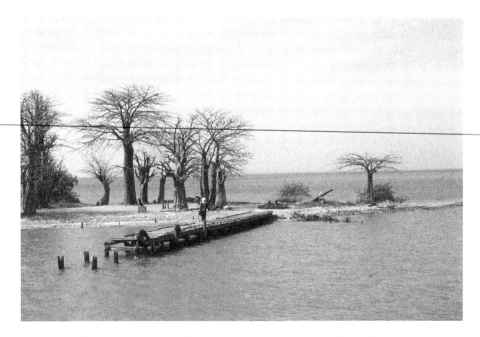

Figure 3.　Ruined fortifications on James Island in the River Gambia.

[4]Gray, *A History, op.cit.*

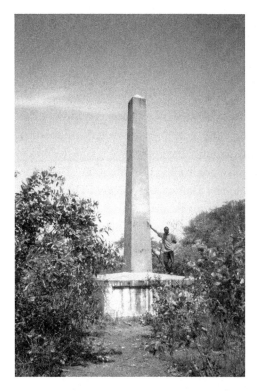 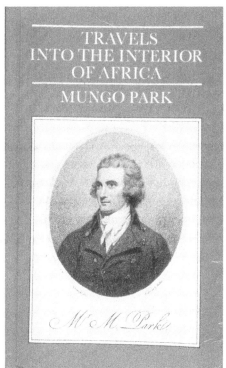

Figure 4. Monument to Mungo Park near the site of Pisania (now abandoned). Mungo Park set out from this spot on two occasions in 1795 and 1805 to walk across West Africa in search of the source of the Nile.

infectious diseases, including intermittent fevers, sleeping sickness and leprosy prevalent in West Africa at that time.[5] On his first expedition, he travelled largely alone but on his second journey he took with him about 50 Europeans only one of whom survived, many dying from febrile illnesses which were almost certainly malaria.

In 1816, the British established a settlement (Bathurst) on an island at the mouth of the river which was later linked to the mainland by a bridge. Mortality among Europeans living in Bathurst was high — a fact commemorated in the persisting name for part of the town as 'half die'. It is likely that most of these deaths were due to malaria or yellow fever. Mortality was also very high among the British traders and missionaries based at Georgetown (now Janjangbureh) on McCarthy Island. By the end of the nineteenth century, improvements in living conditions and the use

---

[5]M. Park, *Travels in the Interior Districts of Africa: Performed in the Years 1795, 1796 and 1797*, John Murray, 1816: London.

of quinine had reduced the risk of death from malaria but this was still high, as noted by Dutton when he visited the Gambia in 1902.[6]

The 1902 Expedition to The Gambia

In 1899, the year after he described the transmission of malaria by mosquitoes, Ronald Ross led an expedition from the recently established Liverpool School of Tropical Medicine and Medical Parasitology to study the epidemiology of malaria in Sierra Leone and to investigate possible ways of controlling this infection.[7] Two years later, a further Liverpool School expedition, led by Dutton, was made to The Gambia. Dutton (Figure 5) died at the age of 29 years from relapsing fever in the Belgian Congo three years after his visit to The Gambia whilst investigating the cause of this disease, and he is remembered through the name, *Borrelia duttoni,* of the spirochaete

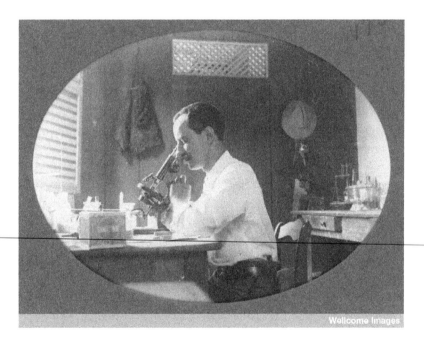

Figure 5. Dr. J. Everett Dutton at his microscope in The Gambia during the expedition which he led to The Gambia in 1902 and during which he identified the cause of Gambian (West African) sleeping sickness. He died in The Congo three years later. (Wellcome Library).

---

[6] J.E. Dutton, Preliminary note upon a trypanosome occurring in the blood of man, *Thompson Yates Laboratory Report,* 1902, **4,** 455–68.

[7] R. Ross, H.E. Annett, E.E. Austen, G.M. Giles and R. Fielding-Ould, *Report of the Malaria Expedition of the Liverpool School of Tropical Medicine and Medical Parasitology,* George Philip & Son, 1900: London.

which is one of the causes of this infection. Although the main purpose of Dutton's visit to The Gambia was the study of malaria, he made another major discovery during his short visit, identifying trypanosomes (*Trypanosoma gambiense*) in the blood of the captain of a Gambian river boat who was thought to have a sleeping sickness and established this as the cause of West African sleeping sickness.[8]

During the course of his visit, Dutton examined the records of patients admitted to the government hospital (now the Royal Victoria Teaching Hospital). He noted that in 1898 there were 23 admissions to hospital among the 63 Europeans living in Bathurst, mainly for malaria, with three deaths including two from blackwater fever. There were a similar number of admissions for malaria among the European population during the following two years, indicating the continuing threat from malaria to the European population of Bathurst.[9] At the time of his visit, a regiment of 108 soldiers from the West Indies, mainly from Barbados, was stationed in Bathurst and he recorded that 10–40 of these relatively malaria naive individuals were admitted to the hospital each month with malaria, with a peak of admissions in September at the height of the rainy season.

During his visit, Dutton undertook a survey of children resident in Bathurst or in a village seven miles outside the capital which was probably Bakau, the site of the present MRC unit. During the survey, he examined each child for enlargement of their spleen and examined their blood for the presence of malaria parasites, the first of many such studies to be done in The Gambia in subsequent years. Dutton found that both the prevalence of malaria parasitaemia and enlargement of the spleen were lower in older children than in younger children (malaria prevalence 82%, 91% and 54% in those aged 0–5, 5–10 and 10–15 years respectively) and he noted that the density of infection was lower in older than in younger children, suggesting that immunity to malaria might develop as a result of repeated infections.[10] The predominant species of malaria parasite detected were *Haemamoeba praecox* (*Plasmodium falciparum*) and *Haemamoeba malariae* (*Plasmodium malariae*). Three infections were recorded as *Haemamoeba vivax* (*Plasmodium vivax*) but these were almost certainly infections with the more prevalent *Plasmodium ovale* which is morphologically very similar to *P. vivax* and which was only recognised as a separate species from the 1920s onwards.

---

[8] J.E. Dutton, Preliminary note upon a trypanosome occurring in the blood of man, *Thompson Yates Laboratory Report*, 1902, **4**, 455–68.

[9] J.E. Dutton and F.V. Theobald, *Report of the Malaria Expedition to The Gambia 1902 of the Liverpool School of Tropical Medicine and Medical Parasitology*, Longmans, Green & Co., 1903: London.

[10] Dutton and Theobald, *Report of the Malaria Expedition, op.cit.*

Dutton collected mosquitoes both on the coast and during a short visit upcountry to McCarthy Island. Most *anopheline* mosquitoes caught on the coast were thought to be *Anopheles costalis* (Loew 1866), a mosquito first described in South Africa. *An. funestus* was the dominant vector on McCarthy Island. Dutton noted that some of the *anophelines* found around Bathurst were able to breed effectively in brackish water, mosquitoes now recognised as *An. melas*, a member of the *An. gambiae* complex. He found *anopheline* mosquitoes breeding in rainwater collecting in boats on the beach, in drains and in small collections of water around households and he made a number of recommendations to the Governor, Sir George Denton, as to how breeding sites could be reduced by removing abandoned boats from the shoreline, clearing drains and covering water containers. These measures were included in an amendment to the Public Health Ordinance, 1887 and some were put into practice.

. The mosquitoes collected by Dutton were made available to the entomologist Theobald who provided a description of these mosquitoes in an appendix to the Dutton report.[11] He confirmed the presence in the collection of *An. costalis*, its darker form *An. costalis* var *melas* and *An. funestus*. *An. costalis* is now considered to be synonymous with *An. gambiae,* first described by Giles,[12] and it is of interest how this mosquito, the most important malaria vector in sub-Saharan Africa where it is widely distributed, acquired its link with The Gambia. In his appendix to the Dutton report, Theobald states 'Col. GILES has described as a distinct species a specimen of *A. costalis* sent me from Gambia by Dr. BUDGETT', which suggests that Giles obtained the specimen which he named as *Anopheles gambiae* from Theobald who had in turn received it from Dr. Budgett, who collected mosquitoes whilst studying fish of the River Gambia. Mattingly reports that the type specimen, now preserved in the British Natural History Museum (Figure 6), was reported in a letter from Budgett to have been collected in a rest house on McCarthy Island,[13] although a recent search could not locate this letter.[14] Subsequent surveys have confirmed the importance of mosquitoes of the *An. gambiae* complex as vectors of malaria in The Gambia.

Following the Liverpool expedition, malaria in The Gambia received little attention outside the country for nearly 50 years. However, examination of annual medical reports to the Governor, covering primarily Bathurst and Georgetown, indicates

---

[11] Dutton and Theobald, *Report of the Malaria Expedition, op.cit.*

[12] G.M. Giles, *A Handbook of the Gnats or Mosquitoes,* John Bale, Sons, and Danielsson, 1902, 2nd ed.: London.

[13] P.F. Mattingly, Names for the *Anopheles gambiae* complex, *Mosquito Systematics,* 1977, **9**, 323–28.

[14] H. Pickering, personal communication.

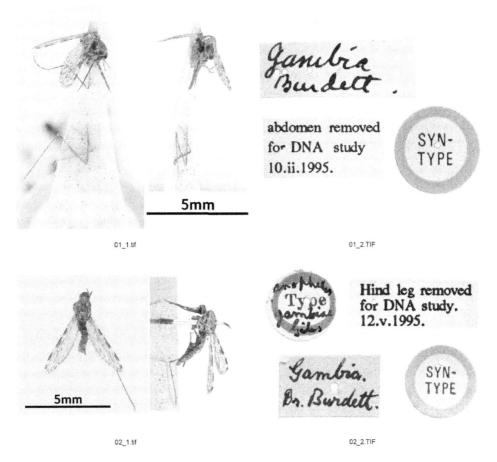

Figure 6. Two mosquitoes held in the entomological collection of the Natural Histroy Museum, London which are the type specimens for *Anopheles gambiae* and which are believed to have been collected on McCarthy Island, The Gambia by Dr. Budgett. (The generous help of Ms TM Howard, Head of Collections, Department of Entomology, The Natural History Museum, London in obtaining these images is acknowledged).

that the incidence of malaria continued to remain high during the first half of the twentieth century with malaria accounting for at least 10% of hospital admissions.[15] In 1947, a large survey was undertaken in 17,000 subjects during which an overall malaria parasite rate of 55% was found. In the 1950s and 1960s, about one half of

---

[15] B.M. Greenwood and H. Pickering, A malaria control trial using insecticide-treated bed nets and targeted chemoprophylaxis in a rural area of The Gambia, West Africa, 1. A review of the epidemiology and control of malaria in The Gambia, West Africa. *Transactions of the Royal Society of Tropical Medicine and Hygiene,* 1993, **87**(Suppl 2), 3–11.

all Gambian children living in rural areas died before the age of five years and it is likely that many of these deaths were due directly or indirectly to malaria.[16]

The Medical Research Council (MRC) Unit, The Gambia

The MRC laboratories

During the Second World War, The Gambia played an important role in supplying troops to fight in North Africa and a military hospital was established on the coast at Fajara, seven miles west of Bathurst. In 1947, this hospital and the accompanying laboratories were taken over by the United Kingdom's Medical Research Council (MRC) as the base for an overseas research unit, which was established the following year. The research unit in The Gambia was one of several research centres in Africa operated by the MRC or the Colonial Office in the final phase of the colonial period, most of which were taken over by national organisations around the time of independence. Because of its small size at the time of independence in 1965 (about 350,000), The Gambia was unable to take on the commitment of supporting the laboratories and they continued to operate in the post-colonial period under the direction of the MRC. The laboratories are still supported financially by the MRC and operated by MRC in collaboration with the Ministry of Health of The Gambia. A new hospital and modern laboratories have been built recently but the original hospital and laboratory buildings are still in use (Figure 7).

The initial research focus of the laboratories, under the leadership of Platt, was nutrition and in 1949 it was decided to study the role of parasites in causing malnutrition. To do this, a survey site was established in the isolated area of West Kiang, then a day's drive from the capital, and in 1950 a comprehensive survey including clinical examination, anthropometry and examination of the population of the village of Keneba was undertaken.[17] (Smith, a nutritionist, was based at the London School of Hygiene and Tropical Medicine [LSHTM] and this study initiated a long-standing collaboration between the MRC unit, The Gambia and LSHTM which continues today). Subsequently, surveys were conducted on a bi-annual or annual basis in Keneba and the neighbouring villages of Jali and Manduar, establishing what would now be known as a demographic surveillance system (DSS), one of the first in Africa. In 1973, the MRC Dunn Nutrition Unit moved its field activities from Uganda to Keneba because of political disturbances

---

[16] W.Z. Billewicz and A. McGregor, The demography of two West African (Gambian) villages, 1951–1975, *Journal of Biological Science,* 1981, **13**, 219–40.

[17] I.A. McGregor and D.A. Smith, A health, nutrition and parasitological survey in a rural village (Keneba) in West Kiang, Gambia, *Transactions of the Royal Society of Tropical Medicine and Hygiene,* 1952, **46**, 403–27.

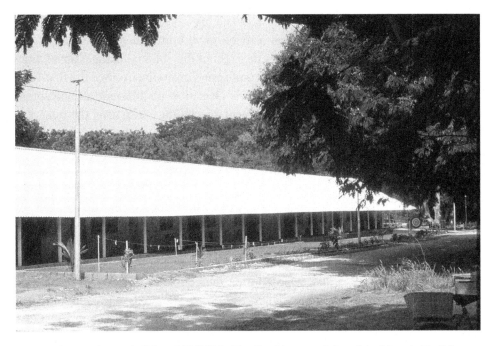

Figure 7. McGregor building, MRC Unit, The Gambia, part of the original hospital buildings.

in Uganda and, in 1980, scientific direction of research at Keneba was taken over by the Dunn Nutrition unit in Cambridge, UK. As a consequence of this change in direction, two new field stations were established in 1982/3 where research on malaria and other infectious diseases could be continued, one at Farafenni on the north bank of the river (this field station was closed in 2009) and the other at Basse in the far eastern part of the country which remains a very active centre for research. In the following sections of this chapter, some of the key findings to emerge from studies on malaria conducted by staff of the MRC unit, The Gambia which have relevance outside the country are summarised.

Malaria entomology

The Gambia has been a site for many pioneering studies on the major vector of malaria in Africa, *An. gambiae*. Three members of the *An. gambiae* complex are found in The Gambia — *An. gambiae sensu stricto, An. arabiensis* and *An. melas*. Little interest was shown in the mosquitoes of The Gambia following the pioneering work of Dutton and Theobald in 1902[18] until 1952, when a survey was made of mosquitoes important to man in rural communities bordering the river and in

---

[18] Dutton and Theobald, *Report of the Malaria Expedition, op.cit.*

peri-urban areas near the coast by Bertram and his colleagues.[19] Thirty years later, Bryan and her colleagues undertook a much more comprehensive survey of the distribution of *anopheline* mosquitoes throughout the country, using a novel morphological approach which recorded chromosomal inversions, one of the first such comprehensive surveys to be carried out.[20] Detection of different chromosomal forms of *An. gambiae s.s.* indicated incipient speciation, illustrating the remarkable plasticity of this vector to occupy different environmental niches. More recently, two different molecular forms of *An. gambiae s.s.* have been identified and these have also been mapped throughout the country.[21]

In the 1960s and 1970s, a number of key studies on the behaviour and ecology of mosquitoes of the *An. gambiae* complex in The Gambia were undertaken by Gillies, Wilkes and Snow and their findings still have relevance to efforts to control this mosquito today. These studies investigated the movement of mosquitoes across the landscape, their ability to detect a host and enter houses, and described the succession of species that occurs during the course of the year in relation to changes in climate and agricultural practices.[22] Since the 1980s, numerous entomological and clinical studies have been carried out to explore the heterogeneity of malaria transmission in The Gambia, illustrating that even within such a small country, transmission of malaria varies markedly in time and place at a range of scales from variations in attractiveness between individuals[23] to marked differences in malaria transmission between villages in the same geographical area.[24]

---

[19] D.S. Bertram, I.A. McGregor and J.A. McFazdean, Mosquitoes of the colony and protectorate of the Gambia, *Transactions of the Royal Society of Tropical Medicine and Hygiene*, 1958, **52**, 135–51.

[20] J.H. Bryan, M.A. Di Deco, V. Petrarca and M. Coluzzi, Inversion polymorphism and incipient speciation in *Anopheles gambiae s.s.* in Gambia West Africa, *Genetica*, 1982, **59**, 167–76.

[21] B. Caputo, D. Nwakanma, M. Jawara, M. Adiamoh, I. Dia, L. Konate, V. Petrarca, D.J. Conway and A. della Torre, *Anopheles gambiae* complex along The Gambia River, with particular reference to the molecular forms of *An. Gambiae s.s.*, *Malaria Journal*, 2008, **7**, 182.

[22] M.T. Gillies and T.J. Wilkes, A comparison of the range of attraction of animal baits and of carbon dioxide for some West African mosquitoes, *Bulletin of Entomological Research*, 1969, **59**, 441–56; M. Gillies and T.J. Wilkes, The vertical distribution of mosquitoes flying over open farmland in The Gambia, *Transactions of the Royal Society of Tropical Medicine and Hygiene*, 1974, **68**, 268–9; W.F. Snow, Mosquito production and species succession from an area of irrigated rice fields in The Gambia, West Africa, *Journal of Tropical Medicine and Hygiene*, 1983, **86**, 237–45; W.F. Snow, Studies of house-entering habits of mosquitoes in The Gambia, West Africa: Experiments with prefabricated huts with varied wall apertures, *Medical and Veterinary Entomology*, 1987, **1**, 9–21.

[23] S.W. Lindsay, J.H. Adiamah, J.E. Miller, R.J. Pleass and J.R. Armstrong, Variation in attractiveness of human subjects to malaria mosquitoes (Diptera: Culicidae) in The Gambia, *Journal of Medical Entomology*, 1993, **30**, 368–73.

[24] C.J. Thomas and S.W. Lindsay, Local-scale variation in malaria infection amongst rural Gambian children estimated by satellite remote sensing, *Transactions of the Royal Socity of Tropical Medicine and Hygiene*, 2000, **94**, 159–63.

Immunity to malaria

The early studies undertaken by McGregor (Figure 8) and his colleagues at Keneba substantiated the epidemiological observations made by Dutton 50 years previously, showing a very high prevalence of malaria parasitaemia and spleno-megaly in children which decreased with increasing age (Figure 9), suggesting that repeated exposure to malaria led to the development of partial immunity to the infection. However, this was not proven and this epidemiological pattern could have been accounted for by less exposure to mosquito bites among adults compared with children. To resolve this issue, McGregor, Cohen and their col-leagues embarked on a courageous experiment in which gamma globulin pre-pared from adult malaria immune Gambians was given to Gambian children with malaria. This led to a slow fall in the parasite count over a period of a few days (Figure 10), proving that gamma globulin obtained from adults contained factors, probably antibodies, capable of impairing multiplication of malaria parasites and thus proving that immunity to malaria could be acquired following

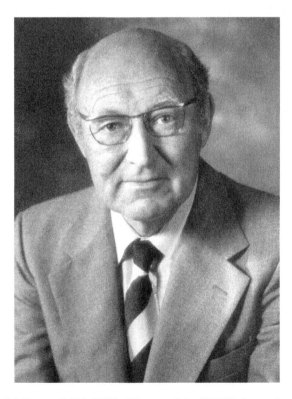

Figure 8. Sir Ian McGregor (1922–2007). Director of the MRC Laboratories, The Gambia from 1954–1974 and from 1979–80. (Photograph courtesy of the Royal Society).

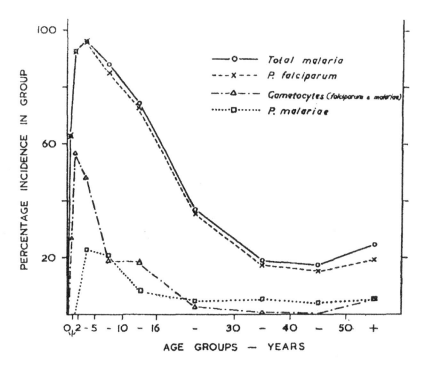

Figure 9.   Prevalence of malaria parasitaemia by age in residents of the Gambian village of Keneba in 1950.[17]

repeated exposure to the parasite.[25] When serum from adult Gambians was given to Tanzanian children with malaria, a similar initial decline in parasitaemia to that seen in Gambian children was observed, but in some children there was a recrudescence in parasitaemia after about four days suggesting that antibodies to malaria had both cross-strain and strain specific components.[26] The nature of the antibodies responsible for this protection of the parasite antigens involved was unknown. Studies conducted in The Gambia in the 1970s by Wilson and his colleagues showed that sera from adult Gambians semi-immune to malaria reacted with a heat stable antigen (S-antigen) present in the sera of Gambian children using a simple precipitation technique. These reactions were highly variable, with some immune sera reacting with some sera obtained from malaria infected children but not with others, one of the first demonstrations of strain

[25] S. Cohen, I.A. McGregor and S. Carrington, Gamma-globulin and acquired immunity to human malaria, *Nature,* 1961, **192**, 733–7.

[26] I.A. McGregor, S.P. Carrington and S. Cohen, Treatment of East African *P. falciparum* malaria with West African human γ globulin, *Transactions of the Royal Society of Tropical Medicine and Hygiene,* 1963, **57**, 170–5.

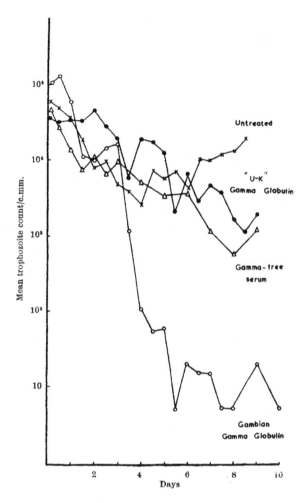

Figure 10. The impact of infusion of gamma globulin obtained from semi-immune adult Gambians on the parasite count of Gambian children with malaria.[25]

specific immune responses to malaria infection.[27] The variability of the antigens involved in this reaction was confirmed in studies undertaken in The Gambia a decade later but the exact nature of the soluble, heat stable S antigens involved in these studies has not been confirmed using modern physicochemical techniques.[28]

---

[27] R.J. Wilson, I.A. McGregor, K. Williams, P.J. Hall and R.K. Bartholomew, Precipitating antibody response to malarial S-antigens, *Transactions of the Royal Society of Tropical Medicine and Hygiene,* 1976, **70**, 308–12.

[28] R.J. Howard, L.J. Panton, K. Marsh, I.T. Ling, E.J. Winchell and R.J. Wilson, Antigenic diversity and size diversity of *Plasmodium falciparum* antigens in isolates from Gambian patients. 1. S-antigens, *Parasite Immunology,* 1986, **8**, 39–55.

As it became clearer that the humoral immune responses to malaria infection were extremely complex, involving antibody responses to many different antigens, an experimental approach was developed at the newly established field station at Farafenni in the early 1980s to try to determine which of the immune responses induced by malaria infection might be most important in providing protection against a new infection. This approach to the study of immunity to malaria involved obtaining samples from a group of children at the beginning of the malaria transmission season, treating the children with an effective antimalarial drug to clear any malaria parasites present at that time, and then following them closely throughout the rainy season to determine who developed malaria and who did not. Correlation of the concentrations of antibodies in the initial serum sample with the subsequent risk of developing malaria provided a way of determining which antibodies were associated with protection against malaria infection, with or without symptoms. Application of this approach led to the demonstration that a group of antibodies that cause agglutination of malaria infected red blood cells was associated with protection against clinical malaria in Gambian children.[29] It was shown subsequently that these antibodies recognise a variant blood stage antigen of *P. falciparum* (PfEMP1) expressed on the surface of infected red blood cells, an antigen which is now known to play a key role in the pathogenesis of severe malaria and of malaria infection of the placenta.[30] Results from a recent study undertaken in The Gambia support the hypothesis that a subset of variant types is associated with severe malaria.[31] Other community cohort studies undertaken in Farafenni and Basse showed that a number of antigens expressed by the merozoite stage of the parasite which are involved in invasion of erythrocytes are also targets of antibodies associated with protection, and that polymorphism in some of these antigens is maintained by immune selection.[32] Subsequent 'treatment-reinfection'

---

[29] K. Marsh, L. Otoo, D.C. Carson and B.M. Greenwood, Antibodies to blood stage antigens of *Plasmodium falciparum* in rural Gambians and their relation to protection against infection, *Transactions of the Royal Society of Tropical Medicine and Hygiene,* 1989, **83**, 293–303.

[30] N.D. Pasternak and R. Dzikowski, PfEMP1: An antigen that plays a key role in the pathogenicity and immune evasion of the malaria parasite *Plasmodium falciparum, International Journal of Biochemistry and Cell Biology,* 2009, **41**, 1463–6.

[31] C.J. Merrick, C. Huttenhower, C. Buckee, A. Amambua-Ngwa, N. Gomez-Escobar, M. Walther, D.J. Conway and M.T. Duraisingh, Epigenetic dysregulation of virulence gene expression in severe *Plasmodium falciparum* malaria, *Journal of Infectious Diseases,* 2012, **205**, 1593–600.

[32] D.J. Conway, D.R. Cavanagh, K. Tanabe, C. Roper, Z.S. Milkes, N. Sakihama, K.A. Bojang, A.M. Oduola, P.G. Kremsner, D.E. Arnot, B.M. Greenwood and J.S. McBride, A principal target of human immunity to malaria identified by molecular population genetic and immunological analyses, *Nature Medicine,* 2000, **6**, 689–92; S.D. Polley, K.K. Tetteh, J.M. Lloyd, O.J. Akpogheneta, B.M. Greenwood, K.A. Bojang and D.J. Conway, *Plasmodium falciparum* merozoite surface protein 3 is a target of allele-specific immunity and alleles are maintained by natural selection, *Journal of Infectious Diseases,* 2007, **195**, 279–87.

studies conducted in several malaria endemic countries have replicated some of these findings, but demonstration of an association does not necessarily mean causation. However, multivariate analyses controlling for confounding variables have helped to identify specific antigens as targets for malaria vaccine development. The long dry season in The Gambia, during which there is virtually no malaria transmission, has enabled informative studies to be conducted on the duration of immune responses to malaria in the absence of re-infection.[33]

All malaria infections can produce the gametocytes required for transmission of malaria infections. Targett, Drakeley and colleagues conducted population studies on the epidemiology of *P. falciparum* gametocytes to determine age-related infectiousness, the importance of asymptomatic infections, and the host factors that influence transmission.[34] Sexual stage immune responses to potential vaccine candidates and to other gametocyte antigens were shown to influence infectivity to mosquitoes in an age-dependent way.[35] The findings from these studies are highly relevant to current national and regional programmes aimed at malaria elimination.

Pathogenesis of malaria

Inoculation of malaria parasites by an infected mosquito may result in an infection which is completely asymptomatic or to one which kills the patient within a few hours of the onset of the illness. Which parasite and host factors determine the outcome of an individual malaria infection are still not completely understood and investigation of risk factors for severe malaria and its pathogenesis has been a focus of research in The Gambia for several decades.[36] Severe malaria may present in several ways but the two most frequent presentations are severe anaemia and cerebral malaria. Early studies conducted in The Gambia focussed on the pathogenesis of malaria anaemia and showed that this has a complex aetiology involving haemolysis of infected red cells, immune damage to non-infected red cells and suppression of

---

[33] O.J. Akpogheneta, N.O. Duah, K.K. Tetteh, S. Dunyo, D.E. Lanar, M. Pinder and D.J. Conway, Duration of naturally acquired antibody responses to blood stage *Plasmodium falciparum* is age dependent and antigen specific, *Infection and Immunity,* 2008, **76**, 1748–55.

[34] C.J. Drakeley, I. Secka, S. Correa, B.M. Greenwood and G.A. Targett, Host haematological factors influencing the transmission of *Plasmodium falciparum* gametocytes to *Anopheles gambiae s.s.* mosquitoes, *Tropical Medicine and International Health,* 1999, **4**, 131–8; C. Drakeley, C. Sutherland, J.T. Bousema, R.W. Sauerwein and G.A. Targett, The epidemiology of *Plasmodium falciparum* gametocytes: Weapons of mass dispersion, *Trends in Parasitology,* 2006, **22**, 424–30.

[35] T. Bousema, C.J. Sutherland, T.S. Churcher, B. Mulder, L.C. Gouagna, E.M. Riley, G.A. Targett and C.J. Drakeley, Human immune responses that reduce the transmission of *Plasmodium falciparum* in African populations, *International Journal of Parasitology,* 2011, **41**, 293–300.

[36] B.Greenwood, K. Marsh and R. Snow, Why do some African children develop severe malaria?, *Parasitology Today,* 1991, **7**, 277–81.

the bone marrow.[37] Studies of the pathogenesis of cerebral malaria showed that tumour necrosis factor (TNF) and other inflammatory cytokines probably play an important role in the pathogenesis of this form of severe malaria.[38] This observation led to a clinical trial of an anti-TNF monoclonal antibody in Gambian children with severe malaria. Although this monoclonal antibody reduced fever, it did not improve the outcome of children with this severe and sometimes fatal condition.[39]

Adherence of malaria infected red blood cells to the endothelium of small blood vessels is believed to play an important role in the pathogenesis of severe malaria and this hypothesis was supported by the results of studies conducted in Gambian children with either uncomplicated or severe malaria, which showed an associa-tion between the ability of parasites to produce clumps of uninfected red cells around an infected red cell (rosettes) with the severity of the disease in the child from whom the parasite was obtained.[40] In contrast, significant differences were not found between parasites obtained from patients with severe or mild disease in the receptors used for invasion of red blood cells.[41]

It is likely that host as well as parasite genetic factors play an important role in determining the severity of an infection with malaria parasites, and to investigate this possibility a large case control study involving over 1,000 Gambian children with severe or uncomplicated malaria and a similar number of uninfected controls was conducted in 1988–90. This study showed that possession of the haemoglobin AS

---

[37] C.A. Facer, R.S. Bray and J. Brown, Direct Coombs antiglobulin reactions in Gambian children with *Plasmodium falciparum* malaria. 1. Incidence and class specificity, *Clinical and Experimental Immunology,* 1979, **35**, 119–12; S. Abdalla, D.J. Weatherall, S.N. Wickramasinghe and M. Hughes, The anaemia of *P. falciparum* malaria, *British Journal of Haematology,* 1980, **46**, 171–83.

[38] D. Kwiatkowski, A.V.S. Hill, I. Sambou, P. Twumasi, J. Castracane, K.R. Manogue, A. Cerami, D.R. Brewster, B.M. Greenwood, TNF concentration in fatal cerebral, non-fatal cerebral, and uncomplicated *Plasmodium falciparum* malaria, *Lancet,* 1990, **336**, 1201–4.

[39] M.B. van Hensbroek, A. Palmer, E. Onyiorah, G. Schneider, S. Jaffar, G. Dolan, H. Memming, J. Frenkel, G. Enwere, S. Bennett, D. Kwiatkowski and B. Greenwood, The effect of a monoclonal antibody to tumour necrosis factor on survival from childhood cerebral malaria, *Journal of Infectious Diseases,* 1996, **174**, 1091–7.

[40] J. Carlson, H. Helmby, A.V. Hill, D. Brewster, B.M. Greenwood and M. Wahlgren, Human cerebral malaria: association with erythrocyte rosetting and lack of anti-rosetting antibodies, *Lancet,* 1990, **336**, 1457–60; C-J. Treutiger, I. Hedlund, H. Helmby, A. Jepson, P. Twumasi, D. Kwiatkowski, J. Carlson, B.M. Greenwood and M. Wahlgren, Rosette formation in *Plasmodium falciparum* isolates and antirosetting activity of sera from Gambians with cerebral or uncomplicated malaria, *American Journal of Tropical Medicine and Hygiene,* 1992, **46**, 503–10.

[41] N. Gomez-Escobar, A. Amambua-Ngwa, M. Walther, J. Okebe, A. Ebonyi and D.J. Conway, Erythrocyte invasion and merozoite ligand gene expression in severe and mild *Plasmodium falciparum* malaria, *Journal of Infectious Diseases,* 2010, **201**, 444–52.

mutation provided a high level of protection against severe malaria and also showed that some histocompatability locus antigens (HLA) were also associated with protection against severe malaria.[42] Exploration of the potential mechanism of one of these HLA associations suggested that it might be mediated through CD8 lymphocyte cytotoxicity directed at liver stages of the infection.[43] Study of genetic risk factors for malaria has continued in The Gambia through participation of the MRC unit in the Malaria Genomic Epidemiology Network (MalariaGEN) (www.malariagen.net) which is studying how genome variation in human, malaria parasite and *anopheline* mosquito populations affects the biology and epidemiology of malaria. Many different single nucleotide polymorphisms in human genes, especially those involved in cytokine production, have been linked to susceptibility to malaria infection and the severity of the infection, although these associations have not always been replicated across studies. Recently, a genome wide analysis of samples from over 1,000 Gambian children with severe malaria and 15,500 cord blood control blood samples was undertaken.[44] This study illustrated, using the HbS locus as a 'positive control', the analytical challenges and special opportunities for genome wide analyses in African populations, which have greater genetic heterogeneity than those in Europe.

Treatment of malaria

During the early years of the MRC laboratories in The Gambia, a number of studies were undertaken on the efficacy of antifolate antimalarials such as

---

[42] A.V. Hill, C.E. Allsopp, D. Kwiatkowski, N.M. Anstey, P. Twumasi, P.A. Rowe, S. Bennett, D. Brewster, A.J. McMichael and B.M. Greenwood, Common West African HLA antigens are associated with protection from severe malaria, *Nature*, 1991, **352**, 595–600.

[43] A.V. Hill, J. Elvin, A.C. Willis, M. Aidoo, C.E. Allsopp, F.M. Gotch, X.M. Gao, M. Takiguchi B.M. Greenwood, A.R. Townsend, A.J. McMichael and H.C. Whittle, Molecular analysis of the association of HLAB53 and resistance to severe malaria, *Nature*, 1992, **36**, 434–9.

[44] M. Jallow, Y.Y. Teo, K.S. Small, K.A. Rockett, P. Deloukas, T.G. Clark, K. Kivinen, K.A. Bojang, D.J. Conway, M. Pinder, G. Sirugo, F. Sisay-Joof, S. Usen, S. Auburn, S.J. Bumpstead, S. Campino, A. Coffey, A. Dunham, A.E. Fry, A. Green, R. Gwilliam, S.E. Hunt, M. Inouye, A.E. Jeffreys, A. Mendy, A. Palotie, S. Potter, J. Ragoussis, J. Rogers, K. Rowlands, E. Somaskantharajah, P. Whittaker, C. Widden, P. Donnelly, B. Howie, J. Marchini, A. Morris, M. SanJoaquin, E.A. Achidi, T. Agbenyega, A. Allen, O. Amodu, P. Corran, A. Djimde, A. Dolo, O.K. Doumbo, C. Drakeley, S. Dunstan, J. Evans, J. Farrar, D. Fernando, T.T. Hien, R.D. Horstmann, M. Ibrahim, N. Karunaweera, G. Kokwaro, K.A. Koram, M. Lemnge, J. Makani, K. Marsh, P. Michon, D. Modiano, M.E. Molyneux, I. Mueller, M. Parker, N. Peshu, C.V. Plowe, O. Puijalon, J. Reeder, H. Reyburn, E.M. Riley, A. Sakuntabhai, P. Singhasivanon, S. Sirima, A. Tall, T.E. Taylor, M. Thera, M. Troye-Blomberg, T.N. Williams, M. Wilson and D.P. Kwiatkowski, Wellcome Trust Case Control Consortium; Malaria Genomic Epidemiology Network. Genome-wide and fine-resolution association analysis of malaria in West Africa, *Nature Genetics*, 2009, **41**, 657–65.

pyrimethamine.[45] But these were not of immediate clinical relevance as chloroquine was still a safe and highly effective treatment for malaria and remained so for the next 30 years. The Gambia was one of the last countries in Africa to be reached by chloroquine resistant strains of *P. falciparum* but, from 1985 onwards, a number of chloroquine treatment failures were noted and local parasite strains became increasingly resistant to this drug.[46] As such, the search for an alternative treatment became a priority. Drugs based on the plant *Artemisia annua* had proved to be extremely effective in treating resistant parasites in South East Asia but in the 1980s, there had been little experience of the use of this class of drugs in Africa. Therefore, in 1989, a trial of artemether was undertaken in children with severe malaria admitted to the Royal Victoria Hospital, Banjul. After a pilot safety study in children with moderately severe malaria, 43 children with severe malaria were randomised to receive either intramuscular artemether or intramuscular chloroquine. There were only two deaths in children who received artemether but six in children who received chloroquine.[47] A subsequent, larger trial compared artemether with quinine in 576 Gambian children with cerebral malaria, using a novel factorial design which also investigated the effect of an anti-TNF monoclonal, as described above.[48] Once again, there were fewer deaths or neurological sequelae in children who received artemether compared with those who received quinine but differences between groups were not statistically significant. More recently, the Royal Victoria Teaching Hospital contributed patients to an even larger, multicentre trial conducted in 5425 children with severe malaria in nine countries in Africa (AQUAMAT) which demonstrated definitively the superiority of an artemisinin

---

[45] A.B. Laing, Studies on the chemotherapy of malaria. 1. The treatment of overt *falciparum* malaria with potentiating combinations of pyrimethamine and sulphormethoxine or dapsone in The Gambia, *Transactions of the Royal Society of Tropical Medicine and Hygiene*, 1970, **64**, 562–8; A.B. Laing, Studies on the chemotherapy of malaria. II. Pyrimethamine resistance in The Gambia, *Transactions of the Royal Society of Tropical Medicine and Hygiene*, 1970, **64**, 569–80.

[46] A. Menon, L. Otoo, E.A. Herbage, B.M. Greenwood, A national survey of the prevalence of chloroquine resistant *Plasmodium falciparum* malaria in The Gambia, *Transactions of the Royal Society of Tropical Medicine and Hygiene*, 1990, **84**, 638–40.

[47] N.J. White, D. Waller, J. Crawley, F. Nosten, D. Chapman, D. Brewster and B.M. Greenwood, Comparison of artemether and chloroquine for severe malaria in Gambian children, *Lancet,* 1992, **339**, 317–21.

[48] M.B. van Hensbroek, E. Onyiorah, S. Jaffar, G. Schneider, A. Palmer, J. Frenkel, G. Enwere, S. Forck, A. Nusmeijer, S. Bennett, B. Greenwood and D. Kwiatkowski D., A comparison of the effect of artemether and quinine on survival from childhood cerebral malaria, *New England Journal of Medicine*, 1996, **335**, 69–75; M. B. van Hensbroek, A. Palmer, E. Onyiorah, G. Schneider, S. Jaffar, G. Dolan, H. Memming, J. Frenkel, G. Enwere, S. Bennett, D. Kwiatkowski and B. Greenwood, The effect of a monoclonal antibody to tumour necrosis factor on survival from childhood cerebral malaria, *Journal of Infectious Diseases*, 1996, **174**, 1091–7.

(artesunate) over quinine for the treatment of severe malaria in African children.[49] This led to a recommendation from WHO that artesunate should now be the first choice for the management of this condition.

Previous experience of treatment for malaria suggested that if artemisinins were to be used widely for treatment of uncomplicated cases of clinical malaria, they should be used in combination with another antimalarial in order to discourage the emergence and spread of resistant strains. Therefore, in the 1990s, Novartis developed a co-formulated combination of artemether and lumefantrine, then known as CGP 56697, as a first line treatment for uncomplicated malaria. The first trials of this artemisinin combination (ACT) in Africa were undertaken at the MRC unit, The Gambia and at the Ifakara Centre in Tanzania.[50] The drug combination proved to be extremely effective in curing uncomplicated clinical malaria, with rapid clearance of parasites and, under its trade name of Coartem[R], this ACT has become one of the mainstays of treatment of malaria across Africa.

One of the advantages of the artemisinin group of drugs, in addition to their ability to clear parasites rapidly, is that they have an effect on gametocytes and thus have the potential to reduce malaria transmission. Taking advantage of the establishment of an insectary at the Farafenni field station, a series of treatment trials was conducted during the 1990s using the membrane feeding assay. These showed that the blood obtained from a patient treated with an ACT was less likely to transmit infection to a susceptible mosquito than blood obtained from a patient treated with chloroquine or sulphadoxine-pyrimethamine (SP). However, the transmission

---

[49] A.M. Dondorp, C.I. Fanello, I.C. Hendriksen, E. Gomes, A. Seni, K.D. Chhaganlal, K. Bojang, R. Olaosebikan, N. Anunobi, K. Maitland, E. Kivaya, T. Agbenyega, S.B. Nguah, J. Evans, S. Gesase, C. Kahabuka, G. Mtove, B. Nadjim, J. Deen, J. Mwanga-Amumpaire, M. Nansumba, C. Karema, N. Umulisa, A. Uwimana, O.A. Mokuolu, O.T. Adedoyin, W.B. Johnson, A.K. Tshefu, M.A. Onyamboko, T. Sakulthaew, W.P. Ngum, K. Silamut, K. Stepniewska, C.J. Woodrow, D. Bethell, B. Wills, M. Oneko, T.E. Peto, L. von Seidlein, N.P. Day, N.J. White for the AQUAMAT group.(2010), Artesunate versus quinine in the treatment of severe *falciparum* malaria in African Children (AQUAMAT): An open-label, randomized trial, *Lancet*, 2010, **376**, 1647–57.

[50] L. von Seidlein, S. Jaffar, M. Pinder, M. Haywood, G. Snounou, B. Gemperli, I. Gathmann, C. Royce and B.M. Greenwood, Treatment of African children with uncomplicated *falciparum* malaria with a new antimalarial drug, CGP 56697, *Journal of Infectious Diseases*, 1997, **176**, 1113–6; L. von Seidlein, K. Bojang, P. Jones, S. Jaffar, M. Pinder, S. Obaro, T. Doherty, M. Haywood, G. Snounou, B. Gemperli, I. Gathmann, C. Royce, K. McAdam and B.M. Greenwood, A randomized controlled trial of artemether/benflumetol, a new antimalarial, and pyrimethamine sulfadoxine in the treatment of uncomplicated *falciparum* malaria in African children. *American Journal of Tropical Medicine and Hygiene,* 1998, **58**, 638–44; C. Hatz, S. Abdulla, R. Mull, D.Schellenberg, I. Gathmann, P. Kibatala, H.P. Beck, M. Tanner and C. Royce, Efficacy and safety of CGP 56697 (artemether and benflumetol) compared with chloroquine to treat acute *falciparum* malaria in Tanzanian children aged 1–5 years, *Tropical Medicine and International Health*, 1998, **3**, 498–504.

blocking ability of ACTs was not complete,[51] an important observation when the possibility of using an ACT in mass drug campaigns directed at interrupting malaria transmission is being considered.

Chemoprophylaxis

At the time when the MRC Laboratories, The Gambia were established, the value of antimalarials in protecting non-immune travellers against malaria was well recognised but whether they could also be used to protect the resident population of malaria endemic areas was less certain. Thus, in 1954, McGregor and colleagues undertook a pilot study in a group of 52 infants born at Sukuta Health Centre, currently the base for MRC studies on infant vaccination, who were allocated to receive weekly chloroquine or a placebo from birth until the age of 36 months. Children who received chloroquine had less malaria, a higher haemoglobin concentration and lower malaria parasite and spleen rates than control children and they were better nourished.[52] However, the results of this pilot study were not followed up because of concerns that chemoprophylaxis might impair the development of natural immunity and favour the dissemination of drug resistant parasites.

Interest in the potential of chemoprophylaxis to protect children living in malaria endemic areas against the deleterious effects of the infection was reawakened 30 years after the study in Sukuta by the author, when a much larger trial of chemoprophylaxis involving over 3,000 children under the age of seven years was conducted in 41 villages in the Farafenni region of The Gambia. During the period 1982–7, Maloprim[R] (pyrimethamine + dapsone) was given fortnightly during the malaria transmission season by village health workers to about 2,500 children aged 3 months –5 years old, resident in 16 villages. A key feature of this study was that it focussed on the impact of the intervention on morbidity and mortality from malaria rather than on its parasitological effects, and ways were developed for measuring these clinical outcomes which subsequently proved valuable in the

---

[51] G. Targett, C. Drakeley, M. Jawara, L. Von Seidlein, R. Coleman, J. Deen, M. Pinder, T. Doherty, C. Sutherland and G. Walraven and P. Milligan, Artesunate reduces but does not prevent posttreatment transmission of *Plasmodium falciparum* to *Anopheles gambiae, Journal of Infectious Diseases*, 2001, **183**, 1254–59; C.J. Sutherland, R. Ord, S. Dunyo, M. Jawara, C.J. Drakeley, N. Alexander, R. Coleman, M. Pinder, G. Walraven and G.A. Targett, Artesunate reduces but does not prevent post-treatment transmission of *Plasmodium falciparum* to *Anopheles gambiae, Journal of Infectious Diseases,* 2005, **183**, 1254–9.

[52] I.A. McGregor, H.M. Gilles, J.H. Walters, A.H. Davies and F.A. Pearson, Effects of heavy and repeated malaria infections on Gambian infants and children; effects on erythrocytic parasitization., *British Medical Journal*, 1956, **2**, 686–92.

evaluation of other interventions such as bednets and vaccines.[53] Administration of Maloprim[R] reduced clinical attacks of malaria by about 80% and overall child mortality by 34% in the first year of the intervention and these high levels of protection were sustained for a further three to four years.[54] High levels of coverage were obtained in some villages for up to five years.[55] There was a modest but significant increase (rebound) in the incidence of clinical malaria in children who had received chemoprophylaxis from the age of three months until five years of age in the year after chemoprophylaxis was stopped. No increase in mortality was observed but the number of deaths was small.[56] Despite these encouraging results, once again they were not followed up because of concerns about impairment of natural immunity to malaria and drug resistance, with attention moving to bednets as the primary malaria preventative tool. However, following increasing recognition that insecticide treated bednets (ITNs) provide only partial protection against malaria, the potential of seasonal malaria prophylaxis to reduce the burden of malaria has once again come to the fore. Following the results of a trial conducted in Senegal which showed that administration of SP + artesunate to children aged 3–59 months on three occasions at monthly intervals during the height of the malaria transmission season reduced clinical attacks of malaria by 86%,[57] a number of further studies of this approach to malaria control have been undertaken in West Africa in recent years. The results of these trials have confirmed the potential of this approach to malaria control, initially known as intermittent preventive

[53] B.M. Greenwood, A.K. Bradley, A.M. Greenwood, P Byass, K. Jammeh, K. Marsh, S. Tulloch, F.S. Oldfield and R. Hayes, Mortality and morbidity from malaria among children in a rural area of The Gambia, *Transactions of the Royal Society of Tropical Medicine and Hygiene*, 1987, **81**, 478–86.

[54] B.M. Greenwood, A.M. Greenwood, A.K. Bradley, R.W. Snow, P. Byass, R.J. Hayes and A.B.H. N'jie, Comparison of two strategies for control of malaria within a primary health care programme in The Gambia, *Lancet*, 1988, 1, 1121–27; A. Menon, R.W. Snow, P. Byass, B.M. Greenwood, R.J. Hayes, A.B.H. N'jie, Sustained protection against mortality and morbidity from malaria in rural Gambian Children by chemoprophylaxis given by village health workers, *Transactions of the Royal Society of Tropical Medicine and Hygiene*, 1990, **84**, 768–72.

[55] S.J. Allen, R.W. Snow, A. Menon and B.M. Greenwood, Compliance with malaria chemoprophylaxis over a five-year period among children in a rural area of The Gambia, *Journal of Tropical Medicine and Hygiene,* 1990, **93**, 313–22.

[56] B.M. Greenwood, P.H. David, L.N. Otoo-Forbes, S.J. Allen, P.L. Alonso, J.R. Armstrong-Schellenberg, P. Byass, M. Hurwitz, A. Menon and R.W. Snow, Mortality and morbidity from malaria after stopping malaria chemoprophylaxis, *Transactions of the Royal Society of Tropical Medicine and Hygiene*, 1995, **89**, 629–33.

[57] B. Cissé, C. Sokhna, D. Boulanger, J. Milet, E.H. Bâ, K. Richardson, R. Hallet, C. Sutherland, K. Simondon, F. Simondon, N. Alexander, O. Gaye, G. Targett, J. Lines, B.M. Greenwood and J-F. Trape, Seasonal intermittent preventive treatment with artesunate and sulfadoxine-pyrimethamine for prevention of malaria in Senegalese children: a randomized, placebo-controlled, double-blind trail, *Lancet*, 2006, **367**, 659–67.

treatment (IPTc) but now called seasonal malaria chemoprevention (SMC).[58] In 2012, SMC was recommended by the WHO for use in areas of the Sahel and sub-Sahel where malaria transmission is highly seasonal and sufficiently intense to make this a cost effective intervention. A study of SMC undertaken in Basse showed that, in The Gambia, administration of drugs by community health workers was a more effective and more cost effective way of delivering SMC than administration by health centre trekking teams visiting villages on monthly occasions.[59]

Pregnant women are at high risk of malaria and it is now recommended by WHO that all pregnant women resident in an area of stable malaria transmission should receive prophylaxis with SP on at least two occasions during pregnancy. This is usually administered at an antenatal clinic but some women find it difficult to reach an antenatal clinical and one of the early studies undertaken at the Farafenni field station showed that preventive drugs could be given safely and effectively to pregnant women by traditional birth attendants.[60] In order to deliver drugs more effectively in the community, it was also shown that women could be taught to treat febrile illnesses in their children at home safely and effectively with chloroquine,[61] one of the first demonstrations of a widely adopted approach to malaria control currently known as home management or community management.

Vector control

In contrast to the situation in most parts of sub-Saharan Africa, bednets (mosquito nets) have been used widely in The Gambia and in neighbouring Guinea Bissau for many decades, even in relatively poor rural areas. How this came about is not certain but the extensive coastal trade between The Gambia and cities such as Liverpool probably facilitated the importation of netting material and local production of nets which were then taken upcountry by itinerant traders. In addition, nets are an important part of a woman's dowry in some Gambian communities. However, despite the

---

[58] A.L. Wilson and IPTc Taskforce, A systematic review and meta-analysis of the efficacy and safety of intermittent preventive treatment of malaria in children (IPTc), *Public Library of Science One*, 2011, **6**, e16976.

[59] K.A. Bojang, F. Akor, L. Conteh, E. Webb, O. Bittaye, D.J. Conway, M. Jasseh, V. Wiseman, P.J. Milligan and B. Greenwood, Two Strategies for the delivery of IPTc in an area of seasonal malaria transmission in The Gambia: A randomized controlled trial, *Public Library of Science Medicine*, 2011, **8**, e1000409.

[60] B.M. Greenwood, A.M. Greenwood, R.W. Snow, P. Byass, S. Bennett and A.B. Hatib-N'jie, The effects of malaria chemoprophylaxis given by traditional birth attendants on the course and outcome of pregnancy, *Transactions of the Royal Society of Tropical Medicine and Hygiene*, 1989, **83**, 589–94.

[61] A. Menon, D. Joof, K.M. Rowan, B.M. Greenwood, Maternal administration of chloroquine: an unexplored aspect of malaria control, *Journal of Tropical Medicine and Hygiene*, 1988, **91**, 49–54.

widespread use of nets in The Gambia, little attention was paid to their potential as a way of controlling malaria in The Gambia or elsewhere until the 1980s. Although it was generally assumed that nets were effective in preventing malaria, there was little evidence to show that this was the case. Thus, in 1982, a systematic survey of the association between the use of bednets (untreated) and the prevalence of malaria was undertaken in a group of villages in the Farafenni area of The Gambia. This confirmed the high usage rate (overall about 80%), showed difference in usage between ethnic groups, established some of the reasons why people used nets and showed that the incidence of malaria was lower in people who used a net than in those who did not.[62] However, the latter finding did not prove a causal relationship as net owners could have been wealthier than others and able to protect themselves against malaria in other ways. Thus, a controlled, community randomised trial of bednets was undertaken in a group of Fula hamlets near to Farafenni where bednet usage was lower than in most other rural areas of The Gambia.[63] This showed a 37% reduction in clinical attacks of malaria, a result which was of borderline statistical significance but an encouraging preliminary finding.

At about this time, reports began to appear of small scale, experimental studies of nets treated with the insecticide permethrin, an approach that had been used first in World War 2 using DDT on nets. Thus, two medium sized, randomised, controlled trials were conducted to determine the efficacy of insecticide treated bednets (ITNs) when used under field conditions in The Gambia. In the first trial, the effects of individually treated nets were investigated by treating only 10% of all the nets in a large village and in the second trial, all the nets in the village were treated.[64] In both studies, a significant reduction in clinical attacks of malaria was observed but this was more marked when all the nets in the village were treated rather than just individual nets (63% vs 50%), suggesting the occurrence of a herd effect with protection of people not using an ITN but sleeping close to someone who was, an effect noted in several subsequent studies.

Following on from these encouraging preliminary trials, a much larger community randomised trial was conducted in 1989 in 73 villages in the central part of The

---

[62] A.K. Bradley, B.M. Greenwood, A.M. Greenwood, K. Marsh, P. Byass, S. Tulloch and R. Hayes, Bednets, (mosquito-nets) and morbidity from malaria, *Lancet*, 1986, **2**, 204–7.

[63] R.W. Snow, K.M. Rowan, S.W. Lindsay and B.M. Greenwood, A trial of bed nets (mosquito nets) as a malaria control strategy in a rural area of The Gambia, West Africa, *Transactions of the Royal Society of Tropical Medicine and Hygiene*, 1988, **82**, 212–5.

[64] R.W. Snow, S.W. Lindsay, R.J. Hayes, B.M. Greenwood, Permethrin-treated bednets (mosquito nets) prevent malaria in The Gambia, *Transactions of the Royal Society of Tropical Medicine and Hygiene*, 1988, **82**, 838–42. R.W. Snow, K.M. Rowan and B.M. Greenwood BM, A trial of permethrin-treated bed-nets in the prevention of malaria in Gambian children, *Transactions of the Royal Society of Tropical Medicine and Hygiene*, 1987, **81**, 563–7.

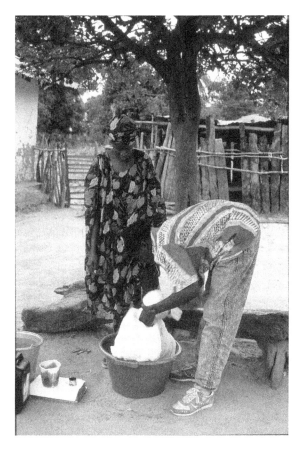

Figure 11.   Treatment of a bed net with insecticide in the community.

Gambia on the south bank of the river, 17 of which were sufficiently large (population > 400 residents) to be part of The Gambia's national primary health care programme. Net ownership was high in these 17 primary health care (PHC) villages.
At the beginning of the malaria transmission season, nearly all the nets in the PHC
villages were dipped in a solution of permethrin under the supervision of a village
health worker (Figure 11). A high rate of coverage was achieved and it was
estimated that over 90% of children slept under a treated net. In addition, chemoprophylaxis with Maloprim[R] was given fortnightly to half the children under six
years of age. Mortality and morbidity from malaria were compared between children who slept under an ITN and those who lived in villages which were too small
to be part of the primary health care programme. Thus, although these smaller
(Non-PHC) villages had similar characteristics to the larger PHC villages, this was
not a strictly randomised, controlled trial. Mortality in PHC and non-PHC villages
was similar immediately prior to the trial but fell dramatically in the PHC villages,
especially in children aged 1–4 years, following the intervention (Figure 12) with

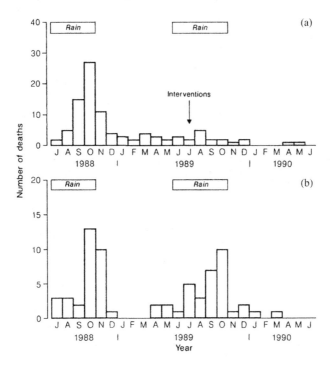

Figure 12. Impact of the combination of insecticide treated bed nets and malaria chemoprophylaxis on mortality in young Gambian children. The seasonal peak in mortality associated with malaria transmission has been almost completely removed.[65]

almost complete abolition of the normal rainy season peak in mortality.[65] Numbers of deaths in children who received Maloprim[R] or placebo were similar but the total number of deaths (19) was small. In contrast, there was a marked additional benefit from adding chemoprophylaxis to the use of ITNs in prevention of clinical attacks of malaria (fever and parasitaemia > 5,000 parasites per μl) with a 97% reduction in incidence as only four clinical attacks were seen in 952 children who received both interventions, illustrating the powerful impact of combining ITNs with chemoprophylaxis. An innovative feature of this trial was that from the beginning, it included an economic and a sociological component. The use of insecticide treated nets was found to be highly cost effective[66] and socially acceptable.[67]

[65] P.L. Alonso, S.W. Lindsay, J.R. Armstrong, M. Conteh, A.G. Hill, P.H. David, G. Fegan, A. de Francisco, A.J. Hall, F.C. Shenton, K. Cham and B.M. Greenwood, The effect of insecticide-treated bednets on mortality of Gambian children, *Lancet*, 1991, **337**, 1499–502.

[66] J. Picard, A. Mills and B.M. Greenwood, The cost effectiveness of chemoprophylaxis with Maloprim® administered by primary health care workers in preventing death from malaria among rural Gambian children less than five years of age, *Transactions of the Royal Society of Tropical Medicine and Hygiene,* 1992, **86**, 580–2.

[67] M.K. Aikins, H. Pickering, P.L. Alonso, U. D'Alessandro, S.W. Lindsay, J. Todd and B.M. Greenwood, A malaria control trial using insecticide-treated bednets and targeted chemoprophylaxis

The findings from this trial encouraged the WHO to support a large scale evaluation of the impact of ITNs in four African countries, studies which confirmed the efficacy of this intervention in reducing overall child mortality by about 20%. In The Gambia, the WHO supported a national implementation programme in which insecticide (but not nets) was provided for free. Evaluation of this programme in five sentinel areas (population 115,895) confirmed the efficacy of ITNs in preventing child deaths which were reduced by 25% in children 1–9 years old.[68] In addition, malaria parasitaemia and low birth weight were less prevalent among primigravidae who slept under an ITN.[69] A high level of insecticide treatment was achieved during this programme when free permethrin was provided but this fell once cost recovery was introduced.[70] In the initial studies, it was necessary to dip untreated nets in insecticide every few months to maintain their efficacy and this proved a challenge to sustainability. However, this problem has been overcome by incorporation of insecticide into the fibre of the netting material to produce long-lasting insecticidal nets (LLINs) which maintain their activity for up to three years and high coverage has been restored in The Gambia following free distribution of LLINs.

In recent years, The Gambia has undertaken some indoor residual spraying with insecticide (IRS) and a trial has recently been completed by the MRC in Upper River Region to determine whether IRS provides any added benefit to high level coverage with ITNs[71] but the results from this trial are not yet available. Attacking larvae rather than adult mosquitoes provides an alternative approach to vector control but this approach was not effective in reducing malaria or anaemia when microbial larvicides were applied by ground teams in the extensive floodplains of

in a rural area of The Gambia, West Africa. 4. Perceptions of the causes of malaria and of its treatment and prevention in the study area, *Transactions of the Royal Society of Tropical Medicine and Hygiene*, 1993, **87** (Suppl 2), 25–30.

[68] U. D'Alessandro, B.O. Olaleye, W. McGuire, P. Langerock, S. Bennett, M.K. Aikins, M.C. Thomson, M.K. Cham, B.A. Cham and B.M. Greenwood, Mortality and morbidity from malaria in Gambian children after introduction of an impregnated bednet programme, Lancet, 1995, **345**, 479–83.

[69] U. D'Alessandro, P. Langerock, S. Bennett, N. Francis, K. Cham and B.M. Greenwood, The impact of national impregnated bednet programme on the outcome of pregnancy in Gambian primigravidae, *Transactions of the Royal Society of Tropical Medicine and Hygiene*, 1996, **90**, 487–92.

[70] M.K. Cham, U. D'Alessandro, J. Todd, S. Bennett, G. Fegan, B.A. Cham and B.M. Greenwood, Implementing a nationwide insecticide-impregnated bednet programme in The Gambia, *Health Policy and Planning*, 1996, **11**, 292–8.

[71] M. Pinder, M. Jawara, L.B. Jarju, B. Kandeh, D. Jeffries, M.F. Llubeeras, J. Mueller, D. Parker, K. Bojang, D.J. Conway and S.W. Lindsay, To assess whether indoor residual spraying can provide additional protection against clinical malaria over current best practice of long-lasting insecticidal mosquito nets in The Gambia: study protocol for a two-armed cluster-randomised trial, *Trials*, 2011, **12**, 147.

the middle reaches of the River Gambia.[72] Failure was probably due to the fact that not all breeding sites could be found and because vectors moved into sprayed areas from neighbouring ones. In this area of The Gambia, aerial spraying might be more successful. House screening without the use of any insecticidal material proved to be a more effective approach with a significant reduction in anaemia, but not parasitaemia, in children less than 10 years old who slept in houses with full screening or just screening of ceilings.[73]

Malaria vaccines

Following the discovery of methods for long term culture of the malaria parasite by Trager and Jensen (1976), one of the first parasites to be put into long term culture came from the MRC laboratories in The Gambia, it was hoped that it might be possible to manufacture a vaccine based on cultured parasites, and preliminary plans were made for a trial of such a vaccine in Keneba in the late 1970s. However, at that time it was not considered safe to use a vaccine based on whole cultured parasites because of the risk of transmitting infections from the human blood used for culture, although this is an approach that has been adopted subsequently in pilot studies in Australia where a low dose of infected red cells has been used successfully and safely as a vaccine.[74] It was another 20 years before the first trial of a malaria vaccine in The Gambia took place.

In the 1980s, a Colombian scientist, Dr. Manuel Patarroyo, developed a malaria vaccine based on three peptides (one of which has been identified as part of the *P. falciparum* merozoite surface protein 1 [MSP1]) known as SPf66. This vaccine gave partial protection against clinical attacks of malaria in trials conducted in Colombia, Ecuador and Brazil. However, it was uncertain whether it would be as effective in areas of Africa where the pressure of infection is much higher than in South America. Thus, Dr. Patarroyo was asked by the author to make his vaccine

---

[72] S. Majambere, M. Pinder, U. Fillinger, D. Ameh, D.J. Conway, C. Green, D. Jeffries, M. Jawara, P.J. Milligan, R. Hutchinson and S.W. Lindsay, Is mosquito larval source management appropriate for reducing malaria in areas of extensive flooding in The Gambia? A cross-over intervention trial, *American Journal of Tropical Medicine and Hygiene*, 2010, **82**, 176–84.

[73] M.J. Kirby, D. Ameh, C. Bottomley, C. Green, M. Jawara, P.J. Milligan, P.C. Snell, D.J. Conway and S.W. Lindsay, Effect of two different house screening interventions on exposure to malaria vectors and on anaemia in children in The Gambia: a randomised controlled trial, *Lancet*, 2009, **374**, 998–1009.

[74] D.J. Pombo, G. Lawrence, C. Hirunpetcharat, C. Rzepczyk, M. Bryden, N. Cloonan, K. Anderson, Y. Mahakunkijcharoen, L.B. Martin, D. Wilson, S. Elliott, S. Elliott, D.P. Eisen, J.B. Weinberg, A. Saul, M.F. Good, Immunity to malaria after administration of ultra-low doses of red cells infected with *Plasmodium falciparum, Lancet*, 2002, **360**, 610–7.

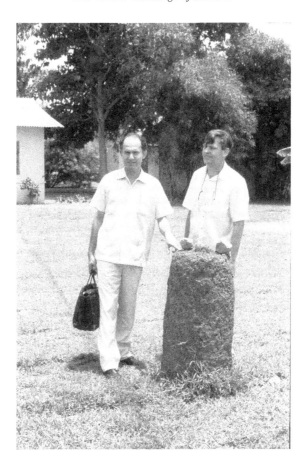

Figure 13. Dr. Patarroyo with the author during a visit to the Gambia in 1990 next to a Gambian standing stone, one of several unearthed during construction of the Farafenni field site.

available for a trial in The Gambia and, after a preliminary visit to The Gambia (Figure 13), he agreed to do so. Unfortunately, the UK Medical Research Council in London did not allow this trial to go ahead on the basis that the product was too experimental, even though it had been approved for trials by the WHO, and so the first African trial of SPf66 was conducted at the Ifakara Centre, Tanzania. In this trial, SPf66 was shown to have 31% (95% CI 0–52%) efficacy against clinical attacks of malaria in children aged 1–5 years.[75] Subsequently, a trial of SPf66 was allowed in The Gambia but this showed no protection against clinical malaria,

---

[75]P.L. Alonso, T. Smith, J.R. Armstrong Schellenberg, H. Masanja, S. Mwankusye, H. Urassa, I. Bastos de Azevedo, J. Chongela, S. Kobero, C. Menendez, N. Hurt, M.C. Thomas, E. Lyimo, N.A. Weiss, R. Hayes, A.Y. Kitua, M.C. Lopez, W.L. Kilama, T. Teuscher, and M. Tanner, Randomised trial of efficacy of SPf66 vaccine against *Plasmodium falciparum* malaria in children in southern Tanzania, *Lancet*, 1994, **344**, 1175–81.

although there was a reduction in the number of strains carried by vaccinated children.[76] Negative results were also obtained in subsequent trials conducted in infants in Tanzania[77] and in older subjects in Thailand[78] and so further development of SPf66 was discontinued. Despite these disappointing results, these trials were important as they established the methods required for the evaluation of malaria vaccines in malaria endemic settings that have been used subsequently in the evaluation of more promising vaccine candidates.

Over a period of many years, the malaria research group at the Walter Reed Army Institute of Medical Research worked on the development of a malaria vaccine based on the circumsporozoite protein (CSP) that covers the surface of the *P. falciparum* sporozoite, first identified at New York University by Nussensweig and her colleagues. Trials with many different variants of this vaccine had only very limited success until a formulation developed at Smith Kline Beecham Biologicals, comprising CSP incorporated into a complex with hepatitis B surface antigen and given with a powerful adjuvant, gave complete protection against an experimental challenge with *P. falciparum* in six of seven American volunteers.[79] These encouraging results led to the initiation of a programme of research to evaluate the potential impact of this vaccine, now known as RTS,S, under conditions of natural challenge. The first trial of RTS,S in a malaria endemic area was conducted in 306 adult residents of Upper River Region of The Gambia in 1998. Vaccine efficacy against malaria infection during the first malaria transmission season after vaccination was 34% overall but protection appeared to wane rapidly after vaccination, being 71% during the first nine weeks

---

[76] U. D'Alessandro, A. Leach, C.J. Drakeley, S. Bennett, B.O. Olaleye, G.W. Fegan, M. Jawara, P. Langerock, M.O. George, G.A.T. Targett and B.M. Greenwood, Efficacy trial of malaria vaccine SPf66 in Gambian infants, *Lancet*, 1995, **346**, 462–7; M. Haywood, D.J. Conway, H. Weiss, W. Metzger, U. D'Alessandro, G. Snounou, G. Targett and B.M. Greenwood, Reduction in the mean number of *Plasmodium falciparum* genotypes in Gambian children immunized with the malaria vaccine SPf66, *Transactions of the Royal Society of Tropical Medicine and Hygiene*, 1999, **93**, (Suppl 1), 65–8.

[77] C.J. Acosta, C.M. Galindo, D. Schellenberg, J.J. Aponte, E. Kahigwa, H. Urassa, J.R. Schellenberg, H. Masanja, R. Hayes, A.Y. Kitua, F. Lwilla, H. Mshinda, C. Menendez, M. Tanner and P.L. Alonso, Evaluation of the SPf66 vaccine for malaria control when delivered through the EPI scheme in Tanzania, *Tropical Medicine and International Health*, 1999, **4**, 368–76.

[78] F. Nosten, C. Luxemburger, D.E. Kyle, W.R. Ballou, J. Wittes, E. Wah, T. Chongsuphajaisiddhi, D.M. Gordon, N.J. White, J.C. Sadoff, D.G. Heppner and the Shoklo SPf66 Malaria Vaccine Trial Group, Randomised double-blind placebo-controlled trial of SPF66 malaria vaccine in children in northwestern Thailand, *Lancet*, 1996, **348**, 701–7.

[79] J.A. Stoute, M. Slaoui, D.G. Heppner, P. Momin, K.E. Kester, P. Desmons, B.T. Wellde, N. Garçon, U. Krzych and M. Marchand, A preliminary evaluation of a recombinant circumsporozoite protein vaccine against *Plasmodium falciparum* malaria. RTS,S Malaria Vaccine Evaluation Group, *New England Journal of Medicine*, 1997, **336**, 86–91.

after vaccination, declining to 0% during the last six weeks of observation.[80] However, efficacy was restored by a booster dose given the following year. Following these encouraging results, a number of age de-escalation studies were conducted in The Gambia which showed that the vaccine was safe and immunogenic in children.[81] Evaluation of RTS,S then moved to Mozambique where it was shown to provide about 50% protection against clinical episodes of malaria both in children aged 1–4 years and in infants when given with EPI vaccines.[82] Following trials which demonstrated the superiority of the AS01 to the AS02 adjuvant, RTS,S/AS01 is now being tested in a large phase 3 trial involving 15,460 infants and children aged 5–17 months recruited in 11 centres in seven countries in Africa, but not The Gambia, with promising initial results in older children with whom approximately 50% protection against uncomplicated and severe malaria was seen during the first year of follow up,[83] although the vaccine has proved less efficacious in young infants.[84]

Although there is a good chance that the current phase 3 trial of RTS,S will show a high enough level of efficacy to warrant its licensure, it is likely to provide only limited protection and more effective second generation vaccines will be needed, which may involve combination of antigens or vaccine constructs.

---

[80]K.A. Bojang, P.J.M. Milligan, M. Pinder, L. Vigneron, A. Alloueche, K.E. Keter, R.W. Ballou, D.J. Conway, W.H.H. Reece, P. Gothard, L. Yamuah, M. DelChambre, G. Voss, B.M. Greenwood, A. Hill, K.P.W.J. McAdam, N. Tornieporth, J.D. Cohen, and T. Dogerty for the RTS, S Malaria Vaccine Trial Team, Efficacy of RTS, S/AS02 malaria vaccine against *Plasmodium falciparum* infection in semi-immune adult men in The Gambia: a randomised trial, *Lancet*, 2001, **358**, 1927–34.

[81]K.A. Bojang, F. Olodude, M. Pinder, O. Ofori-Anyinam, L. Vigneron, S. Fitzpatrick, F. Njie, A. Kassanga, A. Leach, J. Milman, R. Rabinovich, K.P. McAdam, K.E. Kester, D.G. Heppner, J.D. Cohen, N. Tornieporth and P.J. Milligan, Safety and immunogenicity of RTS,S/AS02A candidate malaria vaccine in Gambian children, *Vaccine*, 2005, **14**, 4148–57.

[82]P.L. Alonso, J. Sacarial, J.J. Aponte, A. Leach, E. Macete, J. Milman, I. Mandomando, B. Spiessens, C. Guinovart, M. Espasa, Q. Bassat, P. Aide, O. Ofori-Anyinam, M.M. Navia, S. Corachan, M. Ceuppens, M. C. Dubois, M.A. Demoitié, F. Dubovsky, C. Menéndez, N. Tornieporth, W.R. Ballou, R. Thompson and J. Cohen, Efficacy of the RTS,S/AS02A vaccine against *Plasmodium falciparum* infection and disease in young African children: randomised controlled trial, *Lancet*, 2004, **364**, 1411–20; J.J. Aponte, P. Aide, M. Renom, I. Mandomando, Q. Bassat, J. Sacarial, M.N. Manca, S. Lafuente, A. Barbosa, A. Leach, M. Lievens, J. Vekemans, B. Sigauque, M.C. Dubois, M.A. Demoitié, M. Sillman, B. Savarese, J.G. McNeil, E. Macete, W.R. Ballou, J. Cohen and P.L. Alonso, Safety of the RTS,S/AS02D candidate malaria vaccine in infants living in a highly endemic area of Mozambique: a double blind randomised controlled phase I/IIb trial, *Lancet*, 2007, **370**, 1543–51.

[83]RTS, S Clinical Trials Partnership, First results of phase 3 trial of RTS,S/AS01 malaria vaccine in African children, *New England Journal of Medicine*, 2011, 365, 1683–75.

[84]The RTS, S Clinical Trials Partnership, A phase 3 trial of RTS, S/ASOI malaria vaccine in African infants, *New England Journal of Medicine*, 2012, **376**, 228–95.

Many different constructs are being explored, one of the most promising of which involves the expression of malaria antigens in a viral vector. The Jenner Institute at the University of Oxford is playing a leading role in the development of vaccines using this approach and a number of viral vectored candidate vaccines, including those expressing the CSP protein and the thrombospondin related adhesion protein (TRAP) expressed in modified vaccinia Ankara (MVA), fowl pox and adenovirus vectors have been evaluated in The Gambia.[85] Currently, the latest generation of vectored vaccines including the use of a simian adenovirus and MVA in a prime-boost regimen is being evaluated in Gambian infants with encouraging initial results (Hill, personal communication). These viral vectored vaccines have been shown to be safe and highly effective at inducing strong T cell responses but they have not yet achieved a high enough level of protection against clinical malaria to warrant a phase 3 trial.[86]

Malaria in The Gambia in 2012

During the past decade, increased political and financial support for malaria control has led to a remarkable reduction in the burden of malaria in some but not all countries in sub-Saharan Africa. The Gambia has been one of the countries where success has been achieved with a marked decline in the incidence of malaria

---

[85] V.S. Moorthy, E.B. Imoukhuede, P. Milligan, K. Bojang, S. Keating, P. Kaye, M. Pinder, S.C. Gilbert, G. Walraven, B.M. Greenwood and A.V.S. Hill, A randomised, double-blind, controlled vaccine efficacy trial of DNA/MVA ME-TRAP against malaria infection in Gambian adults, *Public Library of Science Medicine,* 2004, **1**, 128–36.; E.B. Imoukhuede, T. Berthoud, P. Milligan, K. Bojang, J. Ismaili, S. Keating, D. Nwakanma, S. Keita, S. Njie, M. Sowe, S. Todryk, S.M. Laidlaw, M.A. Skinner, T. Lang, S. Gilbert, B.M. Greenwood and A.V. Hill, Safety and immunogenicity of the malaria candidate vaccines FP9 CS and MVA CS in adult Gambian men, *Vaccine,* 2006, **24**, 6526–33; G. A. O'Hara, C.J. Duncan, K.J. Ewer, K.A. Collins, S.C. Elias, F.D. Halstead, A.L. Goodman, N.J. Edwards, A. Reyes-Sandoval, P. Bird, R. Rowland, S.H. Sheehy, I.D. Poulton, C. Hutchings, S. Todryk, L. Andrews, A. Folgori, E. Berrie, S. Moyle, A. Nicosia, S. Colloca, R. Cortese, L. Siani, A.M. Lawrie, S.C. Gilbert and A.V. Hill, Clinical assessment of a recombinant simian adenovirus ChAd63: a potent new vaccine vector, *Journal of Infectious Diseases,* 2012, **205**, 772–81.
[86] E.B. Imoukhuede, L. Andrews, P. Milligan, T. Berthoud, K. Bojang, D. Nwakanma, J. Ismaili, C. Buckee, F. Njie, S. Keita, M. Sowe, T. Lang, S.C. Gilbert, B.M. Greenwood and A.V. Hill, Low-level malaria infections detected by a sensitive polymerase chain reaction assay and use of this technique in the evaluation of malaria vaccines in an endemic area, *American Journal of Tropical Medicine and Hygiene,* 2007, **76**, 486–93.

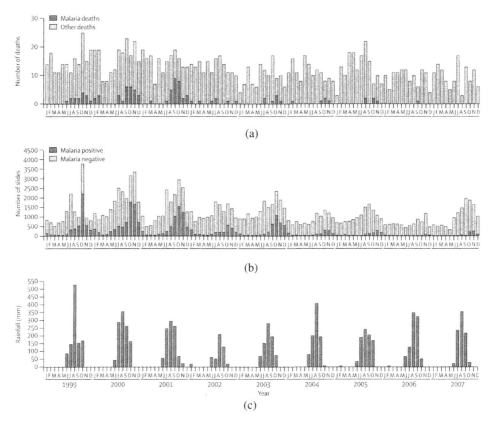

Figure 14. Decline in the incidence of malaria in The Gambia in recent years.[87]

commencing around 2004,[87] (Figure 14) and which contines in the western half of the country.[88] The causes of this decline are not fully understood but probably include a change from chloroquine to SP, and then to an ACT for first line treatment of malaria and a scaling up of the use of LLINs. Better education about malaria and improved access to treatment are likely to have contributed also.

[87] S.J. Ceesay, C. Casals-Pascual, J. Erskine, S.E. Anya, N.O. Duah, A.J. Fulford, S.S. Sesay, I. Abubakar, S. Dunyo, O. Sey, A. Palmer, M. Fofana, T. Corrah, K.A. Bojang, H.C. Whittle, B.M. Greenwood and D.J. Conway, Changes in malaria indices between 1999 and 2007 in The Gambia: a retrospective analysis, *Lancet*, 2008, **372**, 1545–54; S.J. Ceesay, C. Casals-Pascual, D.C. Nwakanma, M. Walter, W, N. Gomez-Escobar, A.J. Fulford, E.N. Takem, S. Nogaro, K.A. Bojang, T. Corrah, M.C. Jaye, M.A. Taal, A.A. Sonko and D.J. Conway, Continued decline of malaria in The Gambia with implications for elimination, *Public Library of Science One*, 2010, **5**, e12242.

[88] S.J. Ceesay, C. Casals-Pascual, D.C. Nwakanma, M. Walther, N. Gomez-Escobar, A.J. Fulford, E.N. Takem, S. Nogaro, K.A. Bojang, T. Corrah, M.C. Jaye, M.A. Toal, A.A. Sonko and D.J. Conway, Continued decline of malaria in The Gambia with implication for elimination, *Public Library of Science One*, 2010, **5**, e12242.

There was a modest increase in the incidence of malaria in Upper River Region in 2010 and 2011, indicating the need for caution, but these encouraging trends have raised interest in the possibility of interrupting malaria transmission in The Gambia. This would almost certainly require additional tools to supplement the existing control programme of ACT treatment, LLINs and IRS, such as the use of mass drug administration (MDA) and/or a vaccine with transmission blocking activity, and would almost certainly have to be carried out in conjunction with The Gambia's neighbours. An initial attempt at MDA in The Gambia was not successful in interrupting transmission but it is probable that a sub-optimal drug combination was used.[89] It would be appropriate if The Gambia, with its long history of contributions to malaria research, was to be one of the first countries in Africa to eliminate this infection.

Conclusion

During the past 100 years, The Gambia, despite its small size and population, has made a more substantial contribution to malaria research than its neighbours and it is of interest to consider why this has been the case. A major factor has been the long-term support provided to the MRC unit in The Gambia by the UK Medical Research Council. This has allowed long term, multi-disciplinary research projects to be conducted, such as the cohort studies conducted in Keneba and Farafenni, which would not have been possible had the investigators needed to rely on short-term project or programme grants. A second key feature has been the sustained support provided to the MRC unit by successive Gambian governments which have put into practice the results of studies undertaken by the unit, such as the early adoption of ITNs and the introduction of *Haemophlius influenzae* type b and pneumococcal conjugate vaccines into the national EPI programme once clinical trials had shown their efficacy. Finally, and most importantly, has been the acceptance by the people of The Gambia that research is essential to improving health, and this has led to their willingness to participate fully in the trials which have been essential to many of the advances described in this chapter.

---

[89] L. von Seidlein, G. Walraven, P.J. Milligan, N. Alexander, F. Manneh, J.L. Deen, R. Coleman, M. Jawara, S.W. Lindsay, C. Drakeley, S. De Martin, P. Olliaro, S. Bennett, M. Schim van der Loeff, K. Okunoye, G.A. Targett, K.P. McAdam, J.F. Doherty, B.M. Greenwood and M. Pinder, The effect of mass administration of sulphadoxine-pyrimethamine combined with artesunate on malaria incidence: a double-blind, community-randomized, placebo-controlled trial in The Gambia, *Transactions of the Royal Society of Tropical Medicine and Hygiene*, 2003, **97**, 217–25.

Acknowledgements

The author thanks Professors Tumani Corrah, Umberto D'Alessandro, Adrian Hill, Dominic Kwiatkowski, Steve Lindsay, Bob Snow and Geoff Targett for their suggestions of topics for inclusion in this review and for their helpful comments on the manuscript.

7 Insecticide–Treated Bednets and Malaria Control: Strategies, Implementation, and Outcome

Harry V. Flaster, Emily Mosites,
and Brian G. Blackburn

Overview

In the global effort to control malaria, insecticide-treated bednets (ITNs) and long-lasting insecticidal nets (LLINs) are among the most effective of the tools available today. Many trials have demonstrated childhood mortality and morbidity reductions with ITN/LLIN use. ITNs protect individuals sleeping under them via the physical barrier they provide, and reduce the number of vectors in communities with high coverage rates through their insecticidal activity. This latter effect may be the primary means by which ITNs/LLINs reduce malaria, and results in protection even to community members not sleeping under them. While conventional ITNs require retreatment with insecticide every six months to remain effective, LLINs do not require retreatment and are designed to remain effective for at least three years under field conditions. Retreatment rates for conventional ITNs are generally too low to sustain effectiveness, and LLINs are more cost-effective than ITNs[1-3]; therefore the World Health Organization (WHO) recommends ITN programs purchase and distribute exclusively LLINs, and that LLIN distribution should focus on achieving high community-wide coverage.

In the past decade, many ambitious goals were set by malaria control organizations, including the 2000 African Summit on Roll Back Malaria in Abuja, Nigeria,

---

[1] A. Tami et al., Evaluation of Olyset insecticide-treated nets distributed seven years previously in Tanzania, *Malaria Journal*, 2004, **3**, 19.

[2] J.A. Schellenberg et al., Re-treatment of mosquito nets with insecticide, *Transactions of the Royal Society of Tropical Medicine and Hygeine*, 2002, **96**(4), 368–9.

[3] P. Guillet et al., Long-lasting treated mosquito nets: a breakthrough in malaria prevention, *Bulletin of the World Health Organisation*, 2001, **79**(10), 998.

which resolved that malaria mortality in Africa would be halved by 2010.[4] Several coverage benchmarks were devised to this end, including >60% coverage of at-risk individuals for malaria (especially pregnant women [PW] and children under five years of age [U5]) with ITNs by 2005.[4] This coverage goal was later revised to >80% ITN coverage of those at-risk for malaria by 2010.[5] In line with these ambitious targets, global funding for malaria control rose dramatically, from $0.3 billion in 2003 to $1.8 billion in 2010.[6] Because ITN/LLIN effectiveness is best when community-wide coverage rates are high, WHO recommends that all individuals in communities endemic for malaria be covered by an LLIN.[6]

While the ambitious Abuja targets for Africa as a whole were not met by 2010, the progress achieved in malaria control during the past decade was substantial. Some nations did meet the Abuja targets and in half of the African countries, >50% of households owned an ITN by 2010, while the proportion of U5s sleeping under an ITN/LLIN was 35% (compared to 17% in 2007, and <5% a decade earlier).[6] Between 2008 and 2010, 289 million ITNs (nearly all of which were LLINs) were distributed in sub-Saharan Africa, enough to cover 76% of the at-risk population. In 2010, a WHO model estimated that 42% of African households owned at least one treated bednet, a substantial increase from only a few years before.[6]

Although the success of ITN/LLIN distribution efforts of the past decade have been encouraging, there must be continued expansion of LLIN distribution to areas with low coverage, development of new insecticides, and increased insecticide resistance surveillance capacity. Continued research and programmatic victories in these areas must occur in order to further malaria control, particularly if regional elimination or even global eradication are to be considered. Reaching these goals would contribute significantly to the aims of the broader Millennium Development Goals set forth by the United Nations in 2000, including Goals 4 and 6 (reduction of U5 mortality by two-thirds, and to halt/decrease the incidence of malaria and other major diseases by 2015).

Parasite and Vector Biology

Malaria is caused by mosquito-borne protozoan parasites and is found throughout much of tropical sub-Saharan Africa, Asia, Oceania, and Latin America. Five

---

[4]World Health Oganization (WHO), The African Summit on Roll Back Malaria (RBM), The Abuja Declaration and the Plan of Action, 2000. Available at: http://www.rbm.who.int/docs/abuja_declaration_final.htm. Accessed on 23 Nov 2011.

[5]RBM partnership, The Global Malaria Action Plan: Key Facts, Figures and Strategies, WHO, 2004, 4: Geneva, Switzerland.

[6]WHO, Global Malaria Programme, World Malaria Report 2010, 2010, 1–60: Geneva, Switzerland.

Plasmodium species cause human malaria: *Plasmodium falciparum, P. vivax, P. ovale, P. malariae*, and *P. knowlesi*. These organisms parasitize human red blood cells and cause hemolytic anemia. In addition to causing over 600,000 annual deaths and 220 million annual symptomatic illnesses globally (primarily among U5s and PW, with 80% in sub-Saharan Africa), malaria is also a common cause of febrile illness in travelers to endemic areas. Manifestations of uncomplicated malaria include fever, anemia, headache, myalgias, arthralgias, and occasionally cough, diarrhea, and hepatosplenomegaly. Severe malaria is usually caused by *P. falciparum* and is characterized by altered mental status, severe anemia, jaundice, hemoglobinuria, renal failure, respiratory distress, shock, hyperparasitemia, and death.

In areas with intense transmission (including much of sub-Saharan Africa), malaria prevalence rates can be ≥80%. In such settings, many infected adults and older children are asymptomatic (or only mildly symptomatic) because of acquired partial immunity. Conversely, U5s and PW are at higher risk of malaria-related morbidity and mortality and bear the brunt of the malaria burden; these individuals are thus referred to as the 'vulnerable population.' Because malaria is transmitted by anophelines, humans can be protected by interventions which prevent mosquito bites, and because *Anopheles* generally bite in the evening and at night, bednets lend themselves well to malaria prevention.

Although our knowledge regarding malaria vectors has increased greatly, many malaria control efforts fail to consider the distribution, species composition, and behavior of local *Anopheles spp.*[7,8] Ignoring these important factors complicates monitoring and evaluation, integration of vector control strategies, and new vector control methods.[9-11]

Among the hundreds of *Anopheles* species, 30–40 are competent malaria vectors. Anophelines are found on every continent except Antarctica. The wide geographic distribution and species variety lead to diverse seasonal and breeding preferences, vector competence, and resting and biting behaviors. These behaviors in turn influence the effectiveness of ITNs/LLINs and other vector-control strategies.

---

[7]A. Enayati and J. Hemingway, Malaria management: past, present, and future, *Annual Review of Entomology*, 2010, **55**, 569–91.

[8]M.E. Sinka *et al.*, The dominant *Anopheles* vectors of human malaria in Africa, Europe and the Middle East: occurrence data, distribution maps and bionomic precis., *Parasites & Vectors*, 2010, **3**, 117.

[9]M. Coetzee, M. Craig and D. le Sueur, Distribution of African malaria mosquitoes belonging to the *Anopheles gambiae* complex, *Parasitology Today*, 2000, **16**(2), 74–7.

[10]J. Utzinger *et al.*, Integrated programme is key to malaria control, *Nature*, 2002, **419**(6906), 431.

[11]L. Alphey *et al.*, Malaria control with genetically manipulated insect vectors, *Science*, 2002, **298**(5591), 119–21.

Among malaria vectors, the *Anopheles gambiae* complex may be the most important globally. This complex consists of seven morphologically indistinguishable species, which are the primary malaria vectors in sub-Saharan Africa. *Anopheles gambiae sensu stricto* is the most efficient and anthropophilic (preferring to feed on humans over animals) species among these vectors.[9,12,13] Two molecular subtypes exist: M, most prevalent in Western Africa and areas with dry seasons and S, more prevalent in Southern Africa and areas with perennial rainfall.[14]

Female anophelines deposit eggs directly onto water, with variables such as vegetation, sunlight preference, degree of urbanization, and other environmental factors influencing this behavior. Larval development takes 5–14 days from hatching. Because vector density is often highest within 300 m of the larval habitat, this habitat is an important variable which affects malaria transmission.[15] Other characteristics which affect vector competence include mosquito density, frequency of human bites, proportion of blood meals from humans (versus animals), feeding interval, extrinsic incubation period, and life expectancy.[16,17]

From the time a female *Anopheles* bites a parasitemic human, *Plasmodium spp.* require 10–21 days to develop within mosquito salivary glands into sporozoites, which are infective to humans. Because only a small proportion of *Anopheles* survive long enough to transmit malaria, any decrease in survivorship can dramatically decrease transmission capacity.

Both adult and larval anophelines are susceptible to insecticides. Certain pyrethroids (synthetically derived chemicals similar to the plant-based toxin, pyrethrin) are approved for vector control through Indoor Residual Spraying (IRS) and application to bednets; pyrethroids can kill mosquitoes on contact. They are also effective as a mosquito deterrent and can temporarily paralyze mosquitoes when a

---

[12]A.K. Githeko *et al.*, Some observations on the biting behavior of *Anopheles gambiae* s.s., *Anopheles arabiensis*, and *Anopheles funestus* and their implications for malaria control, *Experimental Parasitology*, 1996, **82**(3), 306–15.

[13]W. Gu and R.J. Novak, Predicting the impact of insecticide-treated bed nets on malaria transmission: the devil is in the detail, *Malaria Journal*, 2009, **8**, 256.

[14]I.O. Oyewole *et al.*, Behaviour and population dynamics of the major anopheline vectors in a malaria endemic area in southern Nigeria, *Journal of Vector Borne Diseases*, 2007, **44**(1), 56–64.

[15]N. Minakawa, P. Seda and G. Yan, Influence of host and larval habitat distribution on the abundance of African malaria vectors in western Kenya, *American Journal of Tropical Medicine and Hygiene*, 2002, **67**(1), 32–8.

[16]G. MacDonald, *The Epidemiology and Control of Malaria*, Oxford University Press, 1957: Oxford, England.

[17]A.M. Shaukat, J.G. Breman, and F.E. McKenzie, Using the entomological inoculation rate to assess the impact of vector control on malaria parasite transmission and elimination, *Malaria Journal*, 2010, **9**, 122.

sub-lethal dose is encountered (the mosquito "knock-down" effect). The development of mosquito resistance to insecticides is an emerging problem.

ITNs are most effective against mosquitoes that are endophilic (prefer to bite indoors over outdoors), prefer to bite at night over evening/afternoon, and anthropophilic. These biting characteristics vary among species; for example, *An. gambiae* tend to be anthropophilic, endophilic, night-biting mosquitoes, which increases malaria transmission efficiency, but simultaneously makes the species an ideal target for ITN control programs.

An. arabiensis, a primary vector in arid sub-Saharan Africa, feeds on both humans and cattle. In Ethiopia and Zambia, it tends to bite earlier in the evening, limiting the efficacy of ITN/LLIN interventions. Though the species prefers to feed on humans, cattle represent an alternative blood source that allows the species to persist even in populations with high ITN coverage.[18,19]

High ITN coverage in communities endemic for both species can thus result in declines in *An. gambiae* density, with concurrent increases in *An. arabiensis*.[20] ITN and IRS control strategies alone in areas with many *An. arabiensis* mosquitoes may not substantially reduce this vector, which can perpetuate malaria transmission. *An. darlingi*, the major malaria vector in South America, also tends to bite earlier in the evening, and is more likely to bite outdoors than *An. gambiae*. This species (though a less efficient malaria vector than *An. gambiae*) is also less affected by ITNs.[21–24]

---

[18] M. Yohannes and E. Boelee, Early biting rhythm in the afro-tropical vector of malaria, *Anopheles arabiensis*, and challenges for its control in Ethiopia, *Medical and Veterinary Entomology* 2012, **26**(1), 103–5.

[19] I. Tirados *et al.*, Blood-feeding behaviour of the malarial mosquito *Anopheles arabiensis*: implications for vector control, *Medical and Veterinary Entomology*, 2006, **20**(4), 425–37.

[20] M.N. Bayoh *et al.*, *Anopheles gambiae*: historical population decline associated with regional distribution of insecticide-treated bed nets in western Nyanza Province, Kenya, *Malaria Journal*, 2010, **9**, 62.

[21] R. Girod *et al.*, Unravelling the relationships between *Anopheles darlingi* (Diptera: Culicidae) densities, environmental factors and malaria incidence: understanding the variable patterns of malarial transmission in French Guiana (South America), *Annals of Tropical Medicine and Parasitology*, 2011, **105**(2), 107–22.

[22] J.E. Moreno *et al.*, Abundance, biting behaviour and parous rate of anopheline mosquito species in relation to malaria incidence in gold-mining areas of southern Venezuela, *Medical and Veterinary Entomology*, 2007, **21**(4), 339–49.

[23] N.L. Achee *et al.*, Biting patterns and seasonal densities of *Anopheles* mosquitoes in the Cayo District, Belize, Central America with emphasis on *Anopheles darlingi*, *Journal of Vector Ecology*, 2006, **31**(1), 45–57.

[24] A.F. Harris, A. Matias-Arnez and N. Hill, Biting time of *Anopheles darlingi* in the Bolivian Amazon and implications for control of malaria, *Transactions of the Royal Society of Tropical Medicine and Hygiene*, 2006, **100**(1), 45–7.

Changes in mosquito behavior can occur following ITN exposure. In Northern Tanzania, after several years of ITN use, mosquito-biting patterns shifted from late- to earlier evening, when people were less likely to be under an ITN.[25] In Papua New Guinea, *An. farauti* shifted its predominant biting location from indoors to outdoors, biting time to earlier in the evening, and host preference to include non-human species.[26] In Kenya, *An. funestus* and the *An. gambiae* complex shifted biting preference from indoor to outdoor and from later to earlier evening after the introduction of an ITN program.[27,28] These shifts reduce the effectiveness of ITNs.[29] Table 1 enumerates the various points at which the ecological cycles of the vector or parasite can be hindered by ITNs, leading to a collective decrease in malaria transmission.

It is thus crucial to consider the distribution, species composition, behavior, and resistance patterns of local *Anopheles* vectors for malaria control programs. Some anophelines are more susceptible to ITNs than others; for example, *An. funestus* is more susceptible to ITNs than *An. gambiae*, which in turn, is more susceptible than *An. arabiensis*.[30,31] The non-malaria carrying mosquito, *Culex quinquefasciatus*, is more resistant to pyrethroids than anophelines.[30] This intrinsic culicine resistance may indirectly affect the success of ITN programs through a failure of nuisance mosquito reduction, which could negatively impact the perceived effectiveness of ITNs by users. The resistance of culicines to insecticides renders diseases transmitted by these mosquitoes (such as *lymphatic filariasis* and *Japanese encephalitis*) less amenable to vector interventions that depend on pyrethroids, such as ITNs.[32]

[25] N. Braimah *et al.*, Tests of bednet traps (Mbita traps) for monitoring mosquito populations and time of biting in Tanzania and possible impact of prolonged ITN use, *International Journal of Tropical Insect Science*, 2005, **25**(3), 208–13.

[26] H. Bugoro *et al.*, Bionomics of the malaria vector *Anopheles farauti* in Temotu Province, Solomon Islands: issues for malaria elimination, *Malaria Journal*, 2011, **10**, 133.

[27] J.D. Charlwood and P.M. Graves, The effect of permethrin-impregnated bednets on a population of *Anopheles farauti* in coastal Papua New Guinea, *Medical and Veterinary Entomology*, 1987, **1**(3), 319–27.

[28] C.N. Mbogo *et al.*, The impact of permethrin-impregnated bednets on malaria vectors of the Kenyan coast, *Medical and Veterinary Entomology*, 1996, **10**(3), 251–9.

[29] A. Kiszewski *et al.*, A global index representing the stability of malaria transmission, *American Journal of Tropical Medicine and Hygiene*, 2004, **70**(5), 486–98.

[30] K.A. Lindblade *et al.*, Impact of sustained use of insecticide-treated bednets on malaria vector species distribution and culicine mosquitoes, *Journal of Medical Entomology*, 2006, **43**(2), 428–32.

[31] J.E. Gimnig *et al.*, Impact of permethrin-treated bed nets on entomologic indices in an area of intense year-round malaria transmission, *American Journal of Tropical Medicine and Hygiene*, 2003, **68**(4 Suppl), 16–22.

[32] R.T. Rwegoshora *et al.*, Bancroftian filariasis: patterns of vector abundance and transmission in two East African communities with different levels of endemicity, *Annals of Tropical Medicine and Parasitology*, 2005, **99**(3), 253–65.

Table 1: Points of potential disruption of the malaria transmission cycle with ITN use.

Effect of ITN	Outcome on transmission
Vector cannot obtain infected blood meal	Parasite cannot complete lifecycle
Vector cannot transmit parasite to uninfected person	Parasite cannot complete lifecycle
ITN-using human hosts less likely to be parasitized	Decreases overall pool of parasite and therefore vector infection rate
Vector cannot obtain blood meal	Decreased vector parity
Vector cannot rest in preferred location (if indoors)	Decreased vector parity
Vector dies upon contact with insecticide	Vector and parasite cannot complete lifecycle

Bednets: A Historical Perspective

The first bednets were likely designed to avoid nuisance mosquitoes, rather than as preventive measures against vector-borne diseases. The use of bednets dates to the times of Cleopatra (c. 65 BC), but it was not until the 19th century that bednets became more common in Europe and North America.[33] In the United States, the first patent for a bednet was obtained in 1866, and 1897 saw the discovery of *Plasmodium spp.* as the infectious agent of malaria.[34,35] Before the discovery of insecticides, malaria control measures were limited to environmental modifications (such as removing mosquito breeding areas and installing screen doors). In some circumstances, these resulted in successful malaria control, as exemplified by the measures implemented by Gorgas during the construction of the Panama Canal in the early 1900s.[36]

Insecticide-treated bednets (ITNs) were first developed by Russia in the 1930s and then independently by the U.S. during World War II.[37] With the development of synthetic insecticides, it soon became apparent that ITNs could better protect against mosquitoes than untreated bednets. The launch of the WHO Global Malaria Eradication Program in 1955 and resultant global adoption of IRS with the insecticide

---

[33] Horace, Epode, 9.11–16.

[34] The United States Congress, House of Representatives., Executive Documents of the 13th United States Congress, 1867.

[35] Centers for Disease Control and Prevention, The History of Malaria, an Ancient Disease. Available from: http://www.cdc.gov/malaria/about/history. Accessed on 23 Nov 2011.

[36] Centers for Disease Control and Prevention, The Panama Canal. Available from: http://www.cdc.gov/malaria/about/history/panama_canal.html. Accessed on 23 Nov 2011.

[37] S.W. Lindsay and M.E. Gibson, Bednets revisited- old idea, new angle. *Parasitology Today*, 1988, **4**(10), 270–2.

DDT led in part to the potential benefits of ITNs being overlooked. This first eradication effort relied on spraying with DDT, environmental interventions to destroy mosquito breeding sites, and treatment of human malaria cases with chloroquine. This first campaign successfully eliminated malaria throughout much of the developed world, and significantly reduced malaria in areas such as South Asia. However, by 1969 it appeared that this campaign was failing. It did not reach many parts of Africa where malaria is holoendemic, and subsequently, the development of resistance to DDT and concern over environmental effects placed the continued use of insecticides in doubt.

The first ITNs were made from cotton before the discovery that synthetic fibers retained insecticide more avidly. Even with synthetic fibers, conventional ITNs require retreatment every six months to replace insecticide lost through washing and normal wear. In the 1970s, synthetic pyrethroids were developed. Pyrethroids represented a new class of potent insecticides with relatively low toxicity for most vertebrates and fewer environmental effects than DDT, and these compounds renewed interest in ITNs. In 1984, the first successful use of pyrethroid-treated ITNs for malaria control was reported, followed by a 1985 comparison of different pyrethroid insecticides.[38,39]

These preliminary studies sparked a growing interest in this method of malaria prevention, and numerous efficacy trials soon followed.[40] Early studies found that ITNs significantly reduced malaria morbidity and mortality, especially in young children.[41–43] This promising evidence led WHO to adopt ITNs as a cornerstone of the Roll Back Malaria program.[44] The pyrethroid insecticides used included permethrin, deltamethrin, lambdacyhalothrin, and cypermethrin. These insecticides have relatively long residual activity indoors, but break down rapidly under

---

[38]F. Darriet *et al.*, Evaluation of the Efficacy of Permethrin-Impregnated Intact and Perforated Mosquito Nets Against Vectors of Malaria, 1984, 19, WHO/VBC/84.899 WHO: Geneva, Switzerland.

[39]C.F. Curtis and J.D. Lines, Impregnated fabrics against malaria mosquitoes, *Parasitology Today*, 1985, **1**(5), 147.

[40]J.A. Rozendaal, Self-Protection and Vector Control with Insecticide-Treated Mosquito Nets (a Review of Present Status), WHO/VBC/89.965 WHO: Geneva, Switzerland.

[41]P.M. Graves *et al.*, Reduction in incidence and prevalence of *Plasmodium falciparum* in under-5-year-old children by permethrin impregnation of mosquito nets, *Bulletins of the World Health Organisation*, 1987, **65**(6), 869–77.

[42]P.L. Alonso *et al.*, The effect of insecticide-treated bed nets on mortality of Gambian children, *Lancet*, 1991, **337**(8756), 1499–502.

[43]C. Lengeler and R.W. Snow, From efficacy to effectiveness: insecticide-treated bednets in Africa, *Bulletins of the World Health Organisation*, 1996, **74**(3), 325–32.

[44]WHO, RBM, Proposed Methods and Instruments for Situation Analysis, WHO, 1999, 1: Geneva, Switzerland.

exposure to sunlight.[45] Their high specificity for insects and good residual activity on textiles make pyrethroids safe and well suited for use on ITNs and LLINs.[46-49]

In part because of the requirement for retreatment every six months and the poor success of retreatment campaigns, long-lasting insecticidal nets (LLINs) were developed. On these bednets, the insecticide is more stably bound or integrated into the net fabric, obviating the need for retreatment with insecticide. The first LLIN (Olyset) received WHO approval in 2001.[50] LLINs are designed to last at least three years in field-use conditions and retain insecticide for at least twenty washes. LLINs are now the only type of bednet recommended by WHO.[51]

Bednet Materials and Design

Bednets are designed to envelop sleepers in a protective barrier which allows sufficient ventilation and comfort, while denying insects access to the protected space. Although some bednets in use today are made from cotton, most are made from polyester or polyethylene. New materials with mixed fibers are under development.[52]

Netting materials

Cotton bednets were once in widespread use. Because of their inferior strength, insecticide-retention capacity, and flammability characteristics compared to synthetic fibers, cotton bednets are now rarely used.[52]

Polyester bednets are more durable, provide better ventilation, and suffer less insecticide loss than cotton bednets; they are also generally less expensive.

---

[45] W. Takken *et al.*, The experimental application of insecticides from a helicopter for the control of riverine populations of Glossina tachinoides in West Africa: VI. Obervations on Side-effects, *International Journal of Pest Management*, 1978, **24**(4), 455–66.

[46] C. Curtis, Pyrethroid impreganation of bed nets and curtains against malaria mosquitoes, *Pesticide Outlook*, 1990, **1**, 8–11.

[47] K. Naumann, Action of pyrethroids against non-target organisms, in: *Synthetic Pyrethroid Insecticides: Structures and Properties*, Springer-Verlag, 1990, 116–41: Berlin, Germany.

[48] M. Zaim, A. Aitio and N. Nakashima, Safety of pyrethroid-treated mosquito nets, *Medical and Veterinary Entomology*, 2000, **14**(1), 1–5.

[49] S.M. Barlow, F.M. Sullivan, J. Lines, Risk assessment of the use of deltamethrin on bednets for the prevention of malaria, *Food and Chemical Toxicology*, 2001, **39**(5), 407–22.

[50] WHO, Report of the 5th WHOPES Working Group Meeting, WHO, 2001, 4–16: Geneva, Switzerland.

[51] WHO, Global Malaria Programme: Insecticide-treated mosquito nets: a WHO position statement, WHO, 2007: Geneva, Switzerland.

[52] WHO RBM Cabinet Project. Specifications for Netting Materials, WHO, 2001, 5–13: Geneva, Switzerland.

Though polyester bednets are less flammable than cotton, once aflame they can melt and cause severe skin damage. Polyester nets are often textured, which introduces microscopic "frays" into the fibers that soften the net, at the sacrifice of some strength. Because polyester bednets exhibit superior insecticide uptake, they are the WHO-recommended netting material for use in ITN programs which involve regular field-based retreatment.[53]

Nylon bednets have largely been replaced by polyester bednets because nylon is easily soiled, less UV resistant, and lose insecticide more quickly than polyester bednets.

Polyethylene and polypropylene bednets are more durable than polyester, but generally more expensive; some LLINs are made with polyethylene.[54,55] Polypropylene, which is also strong and lightweight, has been used in some recently developed LLINs.

The physical structure of a bednet is an important factor that contributes to efficacy, because holes or tears in netting material allow mosquitoes inside the net. Several standardized measures of bednets have been defined.[56]

Mesh count measures the number of holes/in^2 and by extension, hole size. This determines the smallest insect which a net can exclude. To stop most mosquitoes, bednets must have a minimum mesh count of 156 holes/in^2 (2 mm diameter holes). A mesh count of $\geq$196 is needed to prevent leishmaniasis, which is transmitted by smaller sandflies.[52] The disadvantage of a higher mesh count is decreased ventilation.

Bursting strength measures the capacity of a material to resist rupture by pressure. WHO specifies a minimum bursting strength of 250 kPa, which approximates the force a person applies by grasping the bednet in both hands and pushing the thumbs upward.

Linear Density/Tenacity measures strength per size of net material, or the breaking force measured in gram per unit denier of a yarn or filament. **Denier** is the mass, in grams per 9,000 m yarn, and is characteristic of the netting material (not the finished net itself). The bursting strength is a more useful overall measurement of net strength than denier. Polyethylene and polypropylene nets have a higher denier yarn than polyester nets and are stronger and more durable.[54,56]

[53] WHO, RBM, Insecticide-treated net interventions: A manual for control programme managers, WHO, 2003, 61–3: Geneva, Switzerland.

[54] O. Skovmand and R. Bosselmann, Strength of bed nets as function of denier, knitting pattern, texturizing and polymer, *Malaria Journal*, 2011, **10**, 87.

[55] J.E. Miller, S.W. Lindsay and J.R. Armstrong, Experimental hut trials of bednets impregnated with synthetic pyrethroid or organophosphate insecticide for mosquito control in The Gambia, *Medical and Veterinary Entomology*, 1991, **5**(4), 465–76.

[56] WHO, Technical consultation on specifications and quality control of netting materials and mosquito nets, WHO, 2007, 1–17: Geneva, Switzerland.

Net design

The most common bednet shapes are conical and rectangular. Conical bednets are usually more expensive than rectangular ones because they are sold with a plastic or metal ring.[53] Rectangular bednets provide more sleeping space, but also occupy more area in the home, and require four free corners to hang. A 2009 observational study in Ethiopia found that in round houses typical of that region, it was especially difficult to find four hanging points for rectangular-shaped ITNs. Conical bednets were used 2.3 times more frequently than rectangular ones in this area, although a different survey in Kenya found that rectangular-shaped nets were preferred by 63% of the respondents.[57,58]

Bednets can be designed for either one or multiple sleepers, an important consideration in communities where mothers sleep with young children for the first several years of their lives. Teaching end-users proper bednet usage is an important component of any ITN distribution campaign, and includes points such as:

1) Hanging the ITN from the walls or roof to completely cover the bed or sleeping mat;
2) Tucking the ITN under the mattress during use to prevent mosquito entry;
3) Moving the ITN out of the way during non-use to prevent damage;
4) Ongoing repair of any holes or damage that occur.

Bednets are most commonly available in white, green, and blue. For conventional ITNs, white nets appear to retain insecticide better than green or blue ones, with up to 95% and 89% reductions in deltamethrin uptake in blue and green nets (respectively) compared to white nets.[59] These findings were confirmed by a later study in which a single wash reduced ITN-induced killing of *An. gambiae* in colored ITNs significantly more than in white ITNs.[60] This could be due to low uptake by colored fibers, or high alkalinity on the fibers remaining from the dying process. These shortcomings do not appear to be a problem for colored LLINs.

---

[57] C.A. Baume, R. Reithinger and S. Woldehanna, Factors associated with use and non-use of mosquito nets owned in Oromia and Amhara regional states, Ethiopia, *Malaria Journal*, 2009, **8**, 264.

[58] P.N. Ng'ang'a *et al.*, Bed net use and associated factors in a rice farming community in Central Kenya, *Malaria Journal*, 2009, **8**, 64.

[59] WHO, RBM, Information on Factory Pre-treated Nets and Conventional Treatment of Coloured Mosquito Nets, WHO, 2003, 1–3: Geneva, Switzerland.

[60] S. Duchon *et al.*, Dyeing process may alter the efficacy of insecticide-treated nets, *Journal of Medical Entomology*, 2006, **43**(5), 875–7.

Insecticides

ITNs and LLINs are generally treated with pyrethroid insecticides. Pyrethroids kill many of the mosquitoes that contact the net, have an irritating (excito-repellent) effect on insects which briefly contact ITNs, and can deter mosquitoes (leading to fewer in rooms with an ITN/LLIN present).[61–63]

Six insecticides have passed the WHO Pesticide Evaluation Scheme (WHOPES), a system that monitors the safety and efficacy of insecticides (Table 2). All are pyrethroids, which are preferred because of their safety, repellency, potent knockdown effect, low irritancy, and high efficacy.[48]

Although paresthesias, eye irritation, dizziness, and headache have been noted by individuals treating ITNs (mostly as part of mass campaigns), and eye and nose irritation among ITN users (usually within 24 hours of treatment), field use of pyrethroids poses little serious hazard to those treating or using ITNs. Long-term toxicity studies of pyrethroid insecticides have revealed no teratogenic, carcinogenic, or mutagenic effects in experimental animals, and long-term effects such as these have not been observed in humans.[2, 65] Pyrethroids can be toxic in high concentrations to some aquatic crustaceans and fish; however, there is no evidence that pyrethroids from ITNs are released into aquatic environments in high enough concentrations to harm aquatic life. Pyrethroids also deteriorate rapidly upon exposure to sunlight and therefore have little lasting environmental impact.[45,66]

Little difference has been observed for median knockdown times, mortality, or repellent effects between pyrethroid insecticides. One study showed that bendiocarb 400 mg/m^2, cyfluthrin 30–50 mg/m^2, deltamethrin 15–25 mg/m^2, etofenprox 200 mg/m^2, lambda-cyhalothrin 5–15 mg/m^2, and permethrin 200–500 mg/m^2 did not differ from each other for knockdown or mortality of anophelines, although bendiocarb (a carbamate insecticide), was more effective at killing *Culex*

[61] W. Takken, Do insecticide-treated bednets have an effect on malaria vectors?, *Tropical Medicine and International Health*, 2002, **7**(12), 1022–30.

[62] S.W. Lindsay *et al.*, Pyrethroid-treated bednet effects on mosquitoes of the *Anopheles gambiae* complex in The Gambia, *Medical and Veterinary Entomology*, 1991, **5**(4), 477–83.

[63] F. Chandre *et al.*, Modifications of pyrethroid effects associated with kdr mutation in *Anopheles gambiae*, *Medical and Veterinary Entomology*, 2000, **14**(1), 81–8.

[64] WHO Approved Insecticides for Treatment of Bednets. Available from: http://www.who.int/whopes/Insecticides_ITN_Malaria_ok3.pdf. Accessed on 25 Nov 2011.

[65] J.H. Kolaczinski and C.F. Curtis, Chronic illness as a result of low-level exposure to synthetic pyrethroid insecticides: a review of the debate, *Food and Chemical Toxicology*, 2004, **42**(5), 697–706.

[66] D.P. Weston *et al.*, Aquatic toxicity due to residential use of pyrethroid insecticides, *Environmental Science and Technology*, 2005, **39**(24), 9778–84.

Table 2:   WHO recommended insecticides for treatment of bednets for malaria vector control.

1. Conventional treatments

Insecticide	Formulation	Dosage
Alpha-cypermethrin	SC 10%	20–40 mg/m^2
Cyfluthrin	EW 5%	50 mg/m^2
Deltamethrin	SC 1%, WT 25%, and WT 25% plus binder[1]	15–25 mg/m^2
Etofenprox	EW 10%	200 mg/m^2
Permethrin	EC 10%	200–500 mg/m^2

2. Long-lasting treatments

Product name	Product type	Status of recommendation
ICON® MAXX	Lambda-cyhalothrin 10% CS + binder Target dose of 50 mg/m^2	Interim

SC = suspension concentrate; EW = emulsion, oil in water; WT = water dispersible tablet; EC = emulsifiable concentrate; CS = capsule suspension.

[1] KO TAB 1-2-3.

[2] Milligrams of active ingredient per square meter of netting

Adapted from: WHO Approved Insecticides for Treatment of Bednets.[64]

mosquitoes than the other insecticides tested.[67] However, other data suggest that permethrin may have a better deterrent (but inferior mortality) effect than deltamethrin or alpha-cypermethrin against *An. arabiensis*.[68]

Retreatment of ITNs

Conventional ITNs require retreatment every six months to retain insecticide activity.[50,53,56] They can be treated either at home or a centrally located treatment center, often through mass campaigns. Bednets are treated outdoors and left to dry in the shade.

While only a day's training is required and a team of 2–3 people can treat >200 bednets per day, retreatment rates in Africa have been as low as 5% in

[67]C.F. Curtis, J. Myamba, T.J. Wilkes, Comparison of different insecticides and fabrics for anti-mosquito bednets and curtains, *Medical and Veterinary Entomology*, 1996, **10**(1), 1–11.

[68] F.W. Mosha *et al.*, Comparative efficacies of permethrin-, deltamethrin- and alpha-cypermethrin-treated nets, against *Anopheles arabiensis* and *Culex quinquefasciatus* in northern Tanzania, *Annals of Tropical Medicine and Parasitology*, 2008, **102**(4), 367–76.

some locations just six months after initial distribution.[2,69,70] In Kenya, free ITN retreatment through sentinel dipping stations in communities resulted in 61–67% retreatment rates, but only 7% when villagers were charged for retreatment.[71] The main hindrances to retreatment programs have been logistical issues, cost, and the perception that it is the net itself (rather than the insecticide) that reduces mosquito bites.[3,72] Without insecticide retreatment, ITNs lose their efficacy quickly.

Another challenge with conventional ITNs is their structural integrity over time in field conditions. One study found that the mean number of holes >2 cm in diameter in 75 and 100 denier nets (collected after two years of field use) were 12 and 10, respectively. Overall, 45% of the ITNs were in poor condition (≥7 holes greater than 2 cm in diameter).[73]

Long-lasting insecticidal nets

The low retreatment rates seen in many ITN distribution programs led to the development of ITNs that did not require retreatment. An LLIN is defined by WHO as "a factory-treated mosquito net expected to retain its biological activity for a minimum number of standard WHO washes and a minimum period of time under field conditions." Currently, an LLIN should retain biological activity for at least 20 standard WHO washes and three years of recommended use under field conditions.[74] LLINs are constructed by impregnating bednets with insecticide during the manufacturing process, either by integrating insecticide with the fiber, or by applying a binder that keeps the chemical adherent to the net. These processes render the net more resistant to the loss of the insecticide during its lifespan. LLINs which have insecticide integrated into the netting fibers (vs. application

---

[69]R.K. Dabire *et al.*, Personal protection of long lasting insecticide-treated nets in areas of *Anopheles gambiae* s.s. resistance to pyrethroids, *Malaria Journal*, 2006, **5**, 12.

[70]J. Lines, Review: mosquito nets and insecticides for net treatment: a discussion of existing and potential distribution systems in Africa, *Tropical Medicine and International Health*, 1996, **1**(5), 616–32.

[71]R.W. Snow *et al.*, The effect of delivery mechanisms on the uptake of bed net re-impregnation in Kilifi District, Kenya, *Health policy and planning*, 1999, **14**(1), 18–25.

[72]P.J. Winch *et al.*, Social and cultural factors affecting rates of regular retreatment of mosquito nets with insecticide in Bagamoyo District, Tanzania, *Tropical Medicine and International Health* , 1997, **2**(8), 760–70.

[73]T.E. Erlanger *et al.*, Field issues related to effectiveness of insecticide-treated nets in Tanzania, *Medical and Veterinary Entomology*, 2004, **18**(2), 153–60.

[74]WHO, Guidelines for Laboratory and Field Testing of Long-lasting Insecticidal Mosquito Nets, WHO, 2005, 1: Geneva, Switzerland.

topically with a binder) may require more time for regeneration of insecticide activity after washing.[75] The netting materials of LLINs are also generally more durable than conventional ITNs. WHO now recommends that national malaria control programs purchase and distribute only LLINs.[51,76]

WHOPES Testing: Bednets and other vector control tools must pass a series of laboratory and field tests stipulated by WHOPES before approval for sale to international malaria control organizations. ITNs/LLINs should cause >80% mosquito mortality 24 hours after bednet exposure and/or >95% mosquito knockdown 60 minutes after exposure.[74] ITNs/LLINs are tested against this standard before washing and after each of 20 washes, in both experimental and field settings. Thirteen LLINs have received WHOPES approval; only four (Olyset, Interceptor, PermaNet 2.0 and Yorkool LN) have received full WHO approval, with the remaining LLINs recommended on an interim basis. The number of different LLINs available has grown rapidly in recent years.

The first LLIN to become commercially available and receive full WHO approval was **Olyset**.[50] Olyset is a polyethylene net with wide mesh (4 × 4 mm hole size, 75 holes/inch^2) and 2% permethrin incorporated into the fibers during manufacture. Permethrin diffuses to the surface of the net fibers over time to replace insecticide removed by washing. Olyset LLINs are better ventilated than polyester nets with a narrower mesh, although the wider mesh may allow entry to more mosquitoes than other LLINs.[77] This appears to have impacted efficacy minimally, presumably because the insecticide kills most mosquitoes that travel through the net.[78–80] After washing, diffusion of permethrin to the surface of the net is temperature-dependent and can be accelerated by heating.

The field efficacy of Olyset nets is well established. In rural Tanzania after seven years of continuous use, 100 of 103 randomly selected Olyset LLINs were still

---

[75] J.E. Gimnig *et al.*, Laboratory wash resistance of long-lasting insecticidal nets, *Tropical Medicine and International Health*, 2005, **10**(10), 1022–9.

[76] WHO, Global Malaria Programme, Long-lasting Insecticidal Nets for Malaria Prevention: A Manual for Program Managers, WHO, 2007, 1–9: Geneva, Switzerland.

[77] WHO, WHO Pesticide Evaluation Scheme. Report of the Fifth WHOPES Working Group Meeting, WHO, 2001, 4–16: Geneva, Switzerland.

[78] F.K. Atieli *et al.*, The effect of repeated washing of long-lasting insecticide-treated nets (LLINs) on the feeding success and survival rates of *Anopheles gambiae*, *Malaria Journal*, 2010, **9**, 304.

[79] K. Banek, A. Kilian and R. Allan, Evaluation of interceptor long-lasting insecticidal nets in eight communities in Liberia, *Malaria Journal*, 2010, **9**, 84.

[80] K.A. Lindblade *et al.*, Evaluation of long-lasting insecticidal nets after 2 years of household use, *Tropical Medicine and International Health*, 2005, **10**(11), 1141–50.

in use.[81] The permethrin content was 35% of the original dose and the nets caused a knockdown rate of 92% at 60 minutes, although *Anopheles* mortality was significantly reduced over the lifetime of the net in field conditions, from the reported baseline of 100% to 34%.[1,82] In Côte d'Ivoire, experimental hut trials demonstrated that mortality among *An. gambiae* exposed to Olyset LLINs after three years of use was no different from that seen with new, unused Olyset nets.[83,84] The polyethylene fibers of Olyset nets may be tougher and last longer in the field than typical polyester nets, although it is still uncertain whether Olyset nets can produce consistently high mosquito mortality rates throughout the lifespan of the net. In a 2008 WHOPES supervised multi-country evaluation, a large variation was observed between the countries in terms of bio-efficacy and integrity of Olyset nets.[85]

Like Olyset, **Olyset Plus** is an LLIN made of high-desity mono-filament polyethylene yarn with wide mesh, containing permethrin 2% incorporated into the filaments. In addition, piperonyl butoxide (PBO) 1% is also incorporated into the fibers to act as an insecticide synergist. The addition of PBO provides Olyset Plus with increased activity against pyrethroid-resistant anophelines, and preliminary data suggest Olyset Plus may be superior to Olyset nets even in settings without pyrethroid-resistant vectors.

PermaNet is an LLIN made of warp-knitted multi-filament polyester fibers, with a mesh count of ≥ 156 holes/inch^2 treated with deltamethrin (target concentration 55 mg/m^2) and a binding chemical to keep the insecticide adherent. Compared to Olyset, PermaNets have smaller holes and are less well ventilated; whether this impacts mosquito repellency has not been determined. Although the first-generation PermaNet suffered from quality problems, the second generation PermaNet 2.0 received interim approval by WHOPES in 2001 and full approval in 2009. As with other LLINs, PermaNet 2.0 is designed to remain effective for at least 20 WHO-standardized washes.[84,86,87] A recent multi-country study demonstrated high

[81] R.C. Malima *et al.*, An experimental hut evaluation of Olyset nets against anopheline mosquitoes after seven years use in Tanzanian villages, *Malaria Journal*, 2008, **7**, 38.

[82] T. Jeyalakshmi, R. Shanmugasundaram and P.B. Murthy, Comparative efficacy and persistency of permethrin in Olyset net and conventionally treated net against *Aedes aegypti* and *Anopheles stephensi*, *Journal of the American Mosquito Control Association*, 2006, **22**(1), 107–10.

[83] R. N'Guessan *et al.*, Olyset Net efficacy against pyrethroid-resistant *Anopheles gambiae* and *Culex quinquefasciatus* after 3 years' field use in Cote d'Ivoire, *Medical and Veterinary Entomology*, 2001, **15**(1), 97–104.

[84] J. Hill, J. Lines and M. Rowland, Insecticide-treated nets, *Advances in Parasitology*, 2006, **61**, 77–128.

[85] WHO, WHO Pesticide Evaluation Scheme. Report of the Thirteenth WHOPES Working Group Meeting, WHO, 2009, 1–63: Geneva, Switzerland.

[86] WHO, WHO Pesticide Evaluation Scheme. Report of the Seventh WHOPES Working Group Meeting, WHO, 2003, 29–57: Geneva, Switzerland.

[87] K. Graham *et al.*, Multi-country field trials comparing wash-resistance of PermaNet and conventional insecticide-treated nets against anopheline and culicine mosquitoes, *Medical and Veterinary Entomology*, 2005, **19**(1), 72–83.

efficacy after 20 washes (97% *Anopheles* mortality after a three minute exposure), but the integrity of PermaNets in field conditions over the three year lifespan of the nets requires further evaluation.[75,80,88–92] After obtaining interim approval, sales of PermaNet 2.0 soared and this LLIN now has the largest market share. Several studies have compared PermaNet 2.0 to conventional ITNs and found that they are more durable in the field, retain insecticide longer, and continue to be effective over the course of their three year lifespan.[80,87,88,90,93]

To improve durability, the **PermaNet 2.5** was designed with stronger lower panels. To address pyrethroid resistance, the **PermaNet 3.0** was recently introduced, which incorporates deltamethrin plus a synergistic insecticide [PBO] into the monofilament polyethylene roof, while the side panels have deltamethrin incorporated into polyester. The target deltamethrin concentration is higher than most other LLINs, 180 mg/m^2 on the roof, and 115 mg/m^2 on the sides.[94]

DawaPlus 2.0 is an LLIN with deltamethrin-coated multi-filament polyester fibers. As with PermaNets, a binder is used to ensure the longevity of the insecticide. This binder is the same as that in KO-Tab 1-2-3 (see below). DawaPlus received WHOPES interim approval in 2009.[85]

DuraNet is an LLIN with alpha-cypermethrin incorporated into 150-denier, monofilament, high density polyethylene fibers. Although this LLIN passed the phase one and two initial criteria for WHOPES approval, *Anopheles* mortality dropped below 80% after five washes. DuraNet received an interim WHO recommendation in 2008.

Interceptor is an alpha-cypermethrin coated LLIN. In Benin and Tanzania, Interceptor LLINs resulted in 95% *Anopheles* knockdown after 20 washes, with

[88]K. Gunasekaran and K. Vaidyanathan, Wash resistance of PermaNets in comparison to hand-treated nets, *Acta Tropica*, 2008, **105**(2), 154–7.

[89]M.H. Kayedi, J.D. Lines, and A.A. Haghdoost, Evaluation of the wash resistance of three types of manufactured insecticidal nets in comparison to conventionally treated nets, *Acta Tropical*, 2009, **111**(2), 192–6.

[90]A. Kilian *et al.*, Long-term field performance of a polyester-based long-lasting insecticidal mosquito net in rural Uganda, *Malaria Journal*, 2008, **7**, 49.

[91]F.K. Atieli *et al.*, Wash durability and optimal drying regimen of four brands of long-lasting insecticide-treated nets after repeated washing under tropical conditions, *Malaria Journal*, 2010, **9**, 248.

[92]WHOPES, WHO Recommended Long-lasting Insecticidal Mosquito Nets. http://www.who.int/whopes/Long_lasting_insecticidal_nets_May_2013.pdf. Accessed on 25 Sep 2013.

[93]M.H. Kayedi *et al.*, Entomological evaluation of three brands of manufactured insecticidal nets and of nets conventionally treated with deltamethrin, after repeated washing, *Annals of Tropical Medicine and Parasitology*, 2007, **101**(5), 449–56.

[94]P. Tungu *et al.*, Evaluation of PermaNet 3.0 a deltamethrin-PBO combination net against *Anopheles gambiae* and pyrethroid resistant *Culex quinquefasciatus* mosquitoes: an experimental hut trial in Tanzania, *Malaria Journal*, 2010, **9**, 21.

maximum bioavailability within one day after washing at 25°C.[95,96] Interceptor has received full WHOPES approval.[79]

LifeNet, the only polypropylene LLIN, has deltamethrin incorporated into the 100-denier fibers at a goal concentration of 340 mg/m^2. The manufacturer reports a short insecticide regeneration time between washes for this LLIN.

MAGNet and **Royal Sentry** are two of the newest LLINs available that have interim WHO recommendation. These are polyethylene nets (150 denier yarn, 132 holes/in^2) with alpha-cypermethrin incorporated into the fibers.

NetProtect contains deltamethrin incorporated into polyethylene netting filaments. NetProtect retains 95% *Anopheles* knockdown after 20 washes. Field studies in Tanzania that compared NetProtect to conventional ITNs found that mosquito mortality remained above 80% for NetProtect for 23 washes, whereas ITN mosquito mortality fell below 80% after 17 washes.[97] NetProtect received interim approval in 2009.[85]

Yorkool LN contains deltamethrin coated onto polyester netting. Mosquito knockdown with Yorkool LLINs was >95% for >25 washes, although unwashed Yorkool LNs killed only 55% of mosquitoes after 24 hours during an experimental cone bioassay.[85] However, after being washed 1–20 times, mosquito mortality was consistently higher than the WHO threshold after each wash, nearly 100% during the first 15 washes, and 93% at 20 washes.[85] Yorkool LN has received full WHOPES approval.

One recent study assessed the feeding success and survival rates of *An. gambiae* after exposure to Olyset, PermaNet 2.0, Interceptor, and NetProtect, after repeated washings. No mosquitoes successfully fed after a 10-minute exposure to all four types of unwashed LLINs. However, the feeding success and survival rates increased with the number of washes. After fifteen washes, 61%, 54%, 44%, and 60% of mosquitoes successfully fed through Olyset, PermaNet 2.0, Interceptor, and NetProtect respectively. Twenty-four hour survival rates after 15 washes were 100%, 53%, 82%, and 87% (respectively) after feeding through these nets, suggesting that LLIN effectiveness decreases with washing.[78] A separate study showed that four LLINs (Olyset, PermaNet 2.0, Interceptor, and DawaPlus 2.0), nets dried in the shade retained significantly more insecticide after washing then nets dried in direct sunlight. In addition, LLINs washed by the standard WHO protocol retained significantly more insecticide and were more effective at killing mosquitoes than LLINs washed by

[95] S.K. Sharma *et al.*, Wash-resistance and field evaluation of alphacypermethrin treated long-lasting insecticidal net (Interceptor) against malaria vectors *Anopheles culicifacies* and *Anopheles fluviatilis* in a tribal area of Orissa, India, *Acta Tropical*, 2010, **116**(1), 24–30.

[96] V. Dev *et al.*, Wash resistance and residual efficacy of long-lasting polyester netting coated with alpha-cypermethrin (Interceptor) against malaria-transmitting mosquitoes in Assam, northeast India, *Transactions of the Royal Society of Tropical Medicine and Hygiene*, 2010, **104**(4), 273–8.

[97] WHO, WHO Pesticide Evaluation Scheme. Report of the Eleventh WHOPES Working Group Meeting, WHO, 2008, 9–20: Geneva, Switzerland.

local methods of hand rubbing and beating on rocks; this was consistent across all four brands.[91] Such studies again demonstrate that LLINs while imperfect, retain their mortality and knockdown effects for many washes, an important leap forward from conventional ITNs.[51,87,89,93,98]

Another product, KO Tab 1-2-3, can be used to treat conventional ITNs (or untreated bednets) with an insecticide that appears to be as long-lasting as that found in commercially-produced LLINs. KO Tab 1-2-3 combines deltamethrin with a binding agent that can be applied to conventional bednets through simple dipping and provides a wash-resistant treatment. One study demonstrated that conventional bednets treated with KO Tab 1-2-3 had deltamethrin concentrations and mosquito knockdown rates nearly as high as LLINs even after 30 washes.[99,100] However, a drawback of this method is the poor field durability of many conventional bednets. One study examined ITNs 36 months after distribution and found that 30–40% had either a hole >10 cm in diameter or did not pass the WHO bioassay for killing mosquitoes.[101] Thus, while KO Tab 1-2-3 is an insecticide treatment that can obviate the need for six–month retreatment campaigns for programs that involve conventional bednets, this strategy is limited by the poor durability of conventional bednets, and the ongoing need for repair or replacement.

Other insecticide-treated materials

Pyrethroid-treated curtains, when used to cover all windows of a house, significantly reduced malaria morbidity and all-cause child mortality in Burkina Faso and Kenya.[102,103] In comparison studies, they have proven less effective than ITNs.[104,105]

---

[98] S.K. Sharma *et al.*, Efficacy of permethrin treated long-lasting insecticidal nets on malaria transmission and observations on the perceived side effects, collateral benefits and human safety in a hyperendemic tribal area of Orissa, India, *Acta Tropical*, 2009, **112**(2), 181–7.

[99] A. Yates *et al.*, Evaluation of KO-Tab 1-2-3: a wash-resistant 'dip-it-yourself' insecticide formulation for long-lasting treatment of mosquito nets, *Malaria Journal*, 2005, **4**, 52.

[100] WHO, WHO Pesticide Evaluation Scheme. Report of the Tenth WHOPES Working Group Meeting, WHO, 2007, 37–52: Geneva, Switzerland.

[101] WHO, Global Malaria Programme, World Malaria Report 2009, WHO, 2009, 9–26: Geneva, Switzerland.

[102] A. Habluetzel *et al.*, Insecticide-treated curtains reduce the prevalence and intensity of malaria infection in Burkina Faso, *Tropical Medicine and International Health*, 1999, **4**(8), 557–64.

[103] D.A. Diallo *et al.*, Child mortality in a West African population protected with insecticide-treated curtains for a period of up to 6 years, *Bulletins of the World Health Organisation*, 2004, **82**(2), 85–91.

[104] J.D. Lines, J. Myamba, and C.F. Curtis, Experimental hut trials of permethrin-impregnated mosquito nets and eave curtains against malaria vectors in Tanzania, *Medical and Veterinary Entomology*, 1987, **1**(1), 37–51.

[105] C. Lengeler, Insecticide-treated bed nets and curtains for preventing malaria, *Cochrane Database of Systematic Reviews*, 2004, (2), CD000363.

Table 3: WHO recommended long-lasting insecticidal mosquito nets.

Product name	Product type	Status of WHO recommendation
DawaPlus® 2.0	Deltamethrin coated polyester	Interim
DuraNet®	Alpha-cypermethrin incorporated into polyethylene	Interim
Interceptor®	Alpha-cypermethrin coated polyester	Interim
LifeNet®	Deltamethrin incorporated into polypropylene	Interim
MAGNet™	Alpha-cypermethrin incorporated into polyethylene	Interim
Netprotect®	Deltamethrin incorporated into polyethylene	Interim
Olyset®	Permethrin incorporated into polyethylene	Full
Olyset Plus	Permethrin and PBO incorporated into polyethylene	Interim
PermaNet® 2.0	Deltamethrin coated polyester	Full
PermaNet® 2.5	Deltamethrin coated polyester with strengthened border	Interim
PermaNet® 3.0	Combination of deltamethrin coated on polyester with strengthened border (side panels) and deltamethrin plus piperonyl butoxide incorporated into polyethylene (roof)	Interim
Royal Sentry®	Alpha-cypermethrin incorporated into polyethylene	Interim
Yorkool LN®	Deltamethrin coated on polyester	Full

Adapted from WHO.[92]

Spraying inner surfaces of <u>tents</u> with permethrin or deltamethrin or incorporating such insecticides into plastic sheeting for emergency structures have been effective against indoor-resting mosquitoes. Such practices may offer some coverage for refugee and nomadic populations.[53,106]

<u>Permethrin-treated headscarves and top-sheets</u> in an Afghan refugee camp decreased the incidence of clinical malaria episodes by 64% in children <10 years of age, and by 38% in refugees <20 years of age compared to a placebo group.[107,108] In a Kenyan refugee camp, the use of insecticide-treated clothing reduced malaria incidence by 69% compared to a placebo group (p < 0.001). This approach was culturally acceptable among the refugees and no adverse effects were observed.[109] These materials may be most suitable for complex emergencies involving large populations living in temporary shelters, in which ITN use is impractical.

---

[106] K. Graham *et al.*, Insecticide-treated plastic tarpaulins for control of malaria vectors in refugee camps, *Medical and Veterinary Entomology*, 2002, **16**(4), 404–8.

[107] M. Rowland *et al.*, Permethrin-treated chaddars and top-sheets: appropriate technology for protection against malaria in Afghanistan and other complex emergencies, *Transactions of the Royal Society of Tropical Medicine and Hygeine*, 1999, **93**(5), 465–72.

[108] K. Graham *et al.*, Comparison of three pyrethroid treatments of top-sheets for malaria control in emergencies: entomological and user acceptance studies in an Afghan refugee camp in Pakistan, *Medical and Veterinary Entomology*, 2002, **16**(2), 199–206.

[109] E.W. Kimani *et al.*, Use of insecticide-treated clothes for personal protection against malaria: a community trial, *Malaria Journal*, 2006, **5**, 63.

Insecticide-treated wall coverings are a new methodology currently under study in Africa. These can be an alternative to IRS, and may require replacement only every few years (whereas IRS must be repeated annually). In the context of increasing pyrethroid resistance, alternative insecticides may be used on wall coverings with the added benefit of increased efficacy and reduced resistance.[54,110,111]

Efficacy of untreated bednets

Although untreated bednets are not as effective as ITNs in reducing malaria, they do have some salutary effect on transmission. In the 1980s, two retrospective studies in The Gambia showed that fewer children who regularly slept under untreated bednets developed malaria.[112,113] However, a subsequent randomized controlled trial in The Gambia failed to demonstrate a significant decrease in clinical malaria episodes in children aged 1–9 years who slept under untreated bednets. Following this, interest in untreated bednets for malaria control declined.[114]

A more recent observational study demonstrated fewer clinical malaria episodes among Kenyan children who slept under untreated bednets.[115] These data are supported by comparisons of ITNs to untreated bednets or no nets; a meta-analysis of these trials suggested that bednets alone may be responsible for half of the protective effect of ITNs.[116] Taken together, these studies indicate that untreated bednets do likely have at least some protective effect.

Efficacy of ITNs and LLINs

Experimental hut trials

Data supporting the efficacy of ITNs for the prevention of malaria are robust. An early trial in Tanzania tested permethrin-impregnated bednets and curtains against

---

[110]F. Chandre *et al.*, Field efficacy of pyrethroid treated plastic sheeting (durable lining) in combination with long lasting insecticidal nets against malaria vectors, *Parasites and Vectors*, 2010, **3**(1), 65.

[111]A. Diabate *et al.*, The indoor use of plastic sheeting pre-impregnated with insecticide for control of malaria vectors, *Tropical Medicine and International Health*, 2006, **11**(5), 597–603.

[112]A.K. Bradley *et al.*, Bed-nets (mosquito-nets) and morbidity from malaria, *Lancet*, 1986, **2**(8500), 204–7.

[113]H. Campbell, P. Byass and B.M. Greenwood, Bed-nets and malaria suppression, *Lancet*, 1987, **1**(8537), 859–60.

[114]R.W. Snow *et al.*, A trial of bed nets (mosquito nets) as a malaria control strategy in a rural area of The Gambia, West Africa, *Transactions of the Royal Society of Tropical Medicine and Hygiene*, 1988, **82**(2), 212–5.

[115]T.W. Mwangi *et al.*, The effects of untreated bednets on malaria infection and morbidity on the Kenyan coast, *Transactions of the Royal Society of Tropical Medicine and Hygeine*, 2003, **97**(4), 369–72.

[116]H.W. Choi *et al.*, The effectiveness of insecticide-impregnated bed nets in reducing cases of malaria infection: a meta-analysis of published results, *American Journal of Tropical Medicine and Hygiene*, 1995, **52**(5), 377–82.

An. arabiensis and *An. gambiae* populations in experimental huts fitted with mosquito traps in the 1980s. Compared to untreated bednets, ITNs reduced the number of mosquitoes entering huts by 31%, and the number feeding and surviving by 94%. The protective effect extended to individuals who slept in the same hut as an ITN, even if they did not sleep under one.[104]

Field trials

In Papua New Guinea, two mid-1980s trials demonstrated significant reductions in the incidence and prevalence of *P. falciparum* parasitemia among 0–4 year olds in villages where permethrin-impregnated bednets were distributed.[41,117] A landmark 1991 trial in The Gambia involved permethrin-treated bednet distribution in villages participating in a primary health-care scheme (PHC) at the beginning of the malaria high-transmission season. Over 90% of children in PHC villages slept under ITNs during the study. Compared to villages without this ITN distribution program, overall and malaria-specific mortality in 1–4 year-old children in the intervention villages decreased 37% and 30%, respectively.[42] These dramatic results prompted additional large-scale trials to measure the impact of ITNs on childhood mortality in malaria- endemic areas of Africa.[105]

The most definitive ITN efficacy trial to date has been the Western Kenya ITN Trial, conducted from 1996–1999.[118–123] The study area (near Kisumu, Kenya) was

[117] D.B. Millen, Alternative methods of personal protection against the vectors of malaria in lowland Papua New Guinea with emphasis on the evaluation of permethrin-impregnated bed nets, 1986, MPM thesis, Simon Fraser University, Burnaby, British Columbia, Canada.

[118] P.A. Phillips-Howard *et al.*, The efficacy of permethrin-treated bed nets on child mortality and morbidity in western Kenya I. Development of infrastructure and description of study site, *American Journal of Tropical Medicine and Hygiene*, 2003, **68**(4 Suppl), 3–9.

[119] P.A. Phillips-Howard *et al.*, Efficacy of permethrin-treated bed nets in the prevention of mortality in young children in an area of high perennial malaria transmission in western Kenya, *American Journal of Tropical Medicine and Hygiene*, 2003, **68**(4 Suppl), 23–9.

[120] P.A. Phillips-Howard *et al.*, Impact of permethrin-treated bed nets on the incidence of sick child visits to peripheral health facilities, *American Journal of Tropical Medicine and Hygiene*, 2003, **68**(4 Suppl), 38–43.

[121] S.K. Kariuki *et al.*, Effects of permethrin-treated bed nets on immunity to malaria in western Kenya II. Antibody responses in young children in an area of intense malaria transmission, *American Journal of Tropical Medicine and Hygeine*, 2003, **68**(4 Suppl), 108–14.

[122] S.P. Kachur *et al.*, Maintenance and sustained use of insecticide-treated bednets and curtains three years after a controlled trial in western Kenya, *Tropical Medicine and International Health*, 1999, **4**(11), 728–35.

[123] W.A. Hawley *et al.*, Implications of the western Kenya permethrin-treated bed net study for policy, program implementation, and future research, *American Journal of Tropical Medicine and Hygiene*, 2003, **68**(4 Suppl), 168–73.

holoendemic for malaria and had a *P. falciparum* baseline prevalence of 44% in infants less than six months old, and 83% in children 1–4 years of age. Bednets were used by <5% of the population at baseline.

In the study area, households in half of the villages received enough permethrin-treated ITNs to cover all sleeping spaces ("ITN villages"), while households in the other villages ("control villages") did not receive ITNs during the trial. ITNs were re-treated every six months. About 46,000 ITNs were distributed, for a coverage ratio of 1.34 persons per ITN; 66% of U5s slept under their ITNs as assessed by direct observation.

Field Trials: All-cause childhood mortality

In the Western Kenya trial, crude mortality rates in children 1–59 months of age were significantly lower in ITN villages than control villages over the two year period after ITN distribution (44 vs. 52 per 1,000 child-years). All-cause mortality decreased 16% (95% CI 6–25%) among U5s, 23% among children aged 1–11 months, and 7% among children aged 12–59 months in ITN villages.

Other community-clustered randomized ITN trials (in which villages or geographically defined areas were provided ITNs while matched villages were provided untreated bednets or no nets) have demonstrated mortality benefits approximating this level. In Ghana, all-cause mortality was reduced 17% among U5s who used ITNs in the early 1990s compared to those in villages not given ITNs.[124] In a 1996 trial in Kenya, mortality was reduced 33% among children aged 1–4 years in villages with ITNs compared to those in villages not given ITNs.[125]

Two of the only trials that have examined malaria-specific mortality in children found that malaria-specific death rates decreased less than all-cause mortality.[124,126] Because malaria-specific death rates are difficult to measure, they likely underestimate the true impact of ITNs on mortality; all-cause mortality is likely a more reliable marker of the impact of ITNs.[105]

---

[124]F.N. Binka *et al.*, Impact of permethrin impregnated bednets on child mortality in Kassena-Nankana district, Ghana: a randomized controlled trial, *Tropical Medicine and International Health*, 1996, **1**(2), 147–54.

[125]C.G. Nevill *et al.*, Insecticide-treated bednets reduce mortality and severe morbidity from malaria among children on the Kenyan coast, *Tropical Medicine and International Health*, 1996, **1**(2), 139–46.

[126]U. D'Alessandro *et al.*, Mortality and morbidity from malaria in Gambian children after introduction of an impregnated bednet programme, *Lancet*, 1995, **345**(8948), 479–83.

Field Trials: Malaria morbidity

The Western Kenya ITN Trial also monitored nearly 21,000 U5 sick visits over a four-year period. Compared to before ITN distribution, a significantly greater reduction in all-cause visits to health facilities in ITN villages was seen compared to control villages (37% vs. 10%; p = 0.049). A similar reduction was noted in the number of sick visits ultimately diagnosed as malaria.[120,127]

This study also followed a cohort of 833 children from birth to two years of age to determine the effects of reduced malaria exposure during pregnancy and infancy. In ITN villages (compared to control villages), malaria attack rates in infancy were reduced by 74% and the median time-to-first parasitemia was delayed from 4.5 to 10.7 months (p < 0.001). Notably, the reduced malaria exposure during infancy did not result in higher malaria-related morbidity in one-year-old children. This finding contradicted the previously-held hypothesis that a reduction in mortality from reduced exposure to malaria in the perinatal or infant period would result in less immunity and higher malaria risk in later years.[128–131]

Several studies have reinforced these findings, including a 2002 Tanzanian trial in which 3–4 year-old children who slept under ITNs most of their lives did not experience increased malaria-related morbidity or mortality compared to children who never slept under ITNs.[132] Five-year follow-up data from ITN trials in Burkina Faso and Ghana demonstrated that the survival of children who had slept since birth under an ITN was prolonged compared to children who received an ITN at the end of the trial.[103,133] Although one recent study suggested that the clinical malaria cases in some settings may shift to an older segment of the population (age ≥10 years) 2–3 years after LLIN deployment, taken together, it seems that most likely the "delayed mortality

---

[127] F.O. ter Kuile *et al.*, Impact of permethrin-treated bed nets on malaria, anemia, and growth in infants in an area of intense perennial malaria transmission in western Kenya, *American Journal of Tropical Medicine and Hygiene,* 2003, **68**(4 Suppl), 68–77.

[128] J. Lines and J.R. Armstrong, For a few parasites more: Inoculum size, vector control and strain-specific immunity to malaria, *Parasitology Today,* 1992, **8**(11), 381–3.

[129] R.K. Snow and K. Marsh, Will reducing *P. falciparum* transmission alter malaria mortality among African children?, *Parasitology Today,* 1995, **11**(5), 188–90.

[130] K. Marsh *et al.*, Indicators of life-threatening malaria in African children, *New England Journal of Medicine,* 1995, **332**(21), 1399–404.

[131] R.W. Snow *et al.*, Relation between severe malaria morbidity in children and level of *Plasmodium falciparum* transmission in Africa, *Lancet,* 1997, **349**(9066), 1650–4.

[132] C.A. Maxwell *et al.*, Effect of community-wide use of insecticide-treated nets for 3–4 years on malarial morbidity in Tanzania, *Tropical Medicine and International Health,* 2002, **7**(12), 1003–8.

[133] F.N. Binka *et al.*, Mortality in a seven-and-a-half-year follow-up of a trial of insecticide-treated mosquito nets in Ghana, *Transactions of the Royal Society of Tropical Medicine and Hygeine,* 2002, **96**(6), 597–9.

effect" does not play a significant role in ITN programs, though this remains controversial.[126–139]

ITNs and malaria in pregnancy

Pregnant women and their unborn babies are at high risk of malaria infection, mortality, and morbidity. A review of several trials from Africa and Thailand revealed that ITNs (compared to no bednet use) increased mean birth weight by 55 grams and reduced miscarriages and stillbirths by 33% in a woman's first four pregnancies.[140–143] As parity increases, pregnant women appear to be less susceptible to the most dangerous sequelae of malaria.

Community effect

A key finding of the Western Kenya ITN Trial was the presence of a robust community effect. Reductions in childhood mortality, anemia, and parasitemia in control-village households (without ITNs) approached those seen in ITN-village households, if they were located within 300 meters of a household in an ITN village. The strength of the community effect depended upon the number of nearby compounds with ITNs.

---

[134] J.F. Trape *et al.*, Malaria morbidity and pyrethroid resistance after the introduction of insecticide-treated bednets and artemisinin-based combination therapies: a longitudinal study, *Lancet Infectious Disease*, 2011, **11**(12), 925–32.

[135] U. D'Alessandro and M. Coosemans, Concerns on long-term efficacy of an insecticide-treated bednet programme on child mortality, *Parasitology Today*, 1997, **13**(3), 124–5.

[136] C. Lengeler, J.A. Schellenberg, and U. D'Alessandro, Will reducing *Plasmodium falciparum* malaria transmission alter malaria mortality among African children?, *Parasitology Today*, 1995, **11**(11), 425.

[137] J. Lines, Severe malaria in children and transmission intensity, *Lancet*, 1997, **350**(9080), 813.

[138] L. Molineaux, Nature's experiment: what implications for malaria prevention?, *Lancet*, 1997, **349**(9066), 1636–7.

[139] T. Smith, *et al.*, Associations of peak shifts in age-prevalence for human malarias with bednet coverage, *Transactions of the Royal Society of Tropical Medicine and Hygeine*, 2001, **95**(1), 1–6.

[140] P.W. Gikandi *et al.*, Access and barriers to measures targeted to prevent malaria in pregnancy in rural Kenya, *Tropical Medicine and International Health*, 2008, **13**(2), 208–17.

[141] E.N. Browne, G.H. Maude, and F.N. Binka, The impact of insecticide-treated bednets on malaria and anaemia in pregnancy in Kassena-Nankana district, Ghana: a randomized controlled trial, *Tropical Medicine and International Health*, 2001, **6**(9), 667–76.

[142] C. Gamble *et al.*, Insecticide-treated nets for the prevention of malaria in pregnancy: a systematic review of randomised controlled trials, *Public Library of Science Medicine*, 2007, **4**(3), 107.

[143] C.E. Shulman *et al.*, A community randomized controlled trial of insecticide-treated bednets for the prevention of malaria and anaemia among primigravid women on the Kenyan coast, *Tropical Medicine and International Health*, 1998, **3**(3), 197–204.

These results suggest that the primary effect of ITNs is an area-wide reduction of the mosquito population due to the insecticide, rather than simply the physical barrier protecting individual sleepers. It also suggests that mosquitoes are not simply diverted from ITN-containing households to households without ITNs.[144]

The magnitude of the community effect has important policy implications for ITN distribution. The community effect depends on high ITN coverage, a requirement for impact upon vector populations; there is little evidence for efficacy when ITN coverage is low. The goal of ITN campaigns should therefore be to achieve the highest community-wide coverage possible, to maximize the impact of the community effect.

Most evidence supports the position that the community effect is a more important contributor to the protective capacity of the available ITNs than protection of individual net-enclosed sleepers. A 1987 study in Papua New Guinea demonstrated that ITNs reduced mosquito lifespan and the estimated vector population in ITN villages compared to control villages.[41] A 1988 study in a Burkina Faso village with 100% ITN coverage demonstrated reductions in parous *An. gambiae* and *An. funestus*, resulting in 90% lower inoculation rates and an 82% reduction in malaria incidence, even among non-ITN users in the same village.[145] In a 1991 study in Tanzania, the *Anopheles* population declined after the introduction of ITNs, and sporozoite inoculation rates declined by more than 90%, including people who did not sleep under ITNs.[146]

A subsequent study in Kenya demonstrated that in an area with 90% household ITN coverage, children who did not sleep under an ITN were at a lower risk of developing malaria compared to children who did not sleep under an ITN in control areas (very low ITN coverage). This reduction in malaria incidence occurred if a child in a high-coverage area was up to 1.5 km from the nearest person protected by an ITN.[147] The percentage of children that slept under an ITN the previous night in the immediate area surrounding a child had a greater impact on protection than the child actually sleeping under an ITN.

---

[144] W.A. Hawley *et al.*, Community-wide effects of permethrin-treated bed nets on child mortality and malaria morbidity in western Kenya, *American Journal of Tropical Medicine and Hygiene*, 2003, **68**(4 Suppl), 121–7.

[145] P. Carnevale *et al.*, Control of malaria using mosquito nets impregnated with pyrethroids in Burkina Faso, *Bulletin de la Société de pathologie exotique*, 1988, **81**(5), 832–46.

[146] S.M. Magesa *et al.*, Trial of pyrethroid impregnated bednets in an area of Tanzania holoendemic for malaria. Part 2. Effects on the malaria vector population, *Acta Tropical*, 1991, **49**(2), 97–108.

[147] S.C. Howard *et al.*, Evidence for a mass community effect of insecticide-treated bednets on the incidence of malaria on the Kenyan coast, *Transactions of the Royal Society of Tropical Medicine and Hygeine*, 2000, **94**(4), 357–60.

A 2002 study in Tanzania demonstrated that even among those not sleeping under ITNs, children aged 6–24 months in villages with high ITN coverage were bitten 90–95% less frequently by anophelines and suffered 55–75% fewer malaria episodes than children in villages with low ITN coverage.[132] Another recent study in Ghana found that among children aged 6–60 months without ITNs, hemoglobin levels were higher if they lived within 300 m of a household with an ITN than if they lived >300 m from any households with ITNs.[148]

Taken together, the current evidence favors high community-wide ITN/LLIN coverage, rather than distribution limited only to vulnerable groups. This conclusion is consistent with the entomologic and demographic characteristics of much of the developing world where malaria is holoendemic. In these settings, adults and children over five years of age constitute the bulk of the population and >80% of human-to-mosquito transmission.[149] Targeting only 20% of transmission while leaving the remaining 80% of the population unprotected is unlikely to achieve the same protective effect as targeting the entire population and would adversely impact the community effect on vector populations. The counter-argument to this is that most morbidity and mortality occurs in the U5/PW population, and focusing coverage on only these individuals allows larger geographic areas to be addressed. Further study is needed in this regard, including comparisons of more widespread initial geographic coverage limited to U5/PW vs. narrower coverage of entire populations; modeling of the effect of different coverage levels on a more robust scale would also be useful.

For now, given that most ITN field trials have been conducted using high community-wide ITN coverage levels, and have targeted entire communities rather than just vulnerable individuals, it seems advisable for most ITN/LLIN distribution programs to strive for high community-wide coverage, even if this means targeting a smaller geographic area initially.[105,144,147,150] In recognition of the growing evidence for the community effect from ITN/LLIN distribution, WHO recently recommended that national malaria control programs should distribute LLINs with the goal of achieving high community-wide coverage.[51]

---

[148] E. Klinkenberg *et al.*, Cohort trial reveals community impact of insecticide-treated nets on malariometric indices in urban Ghana, *Transactions of the Royal Society of Tropical Medicine and Hygiene*, 2010, **104**(7), 496–503.

[149] A. Ross, G. Killeen and T. Smith, Relationships between host infectivity to mosquitoes and asexual parasite density in *Plasmodium falciparum*, *American Journal of Tropical Medicine and Hygiene*, 2006, **75**(2 Suppl), 32–7.

[150] L. Gosoniu *et al.*, Spatial effects of mosquito bednets on child mortality, *BMC Public Health*, 2008, **8**, 356.

LLINs

Most field trials involving LLINs have demonstrated similar protective efficacy against malaria as the above trials involving conventional ITNs. Although large-scale field trials involving LLINs are currently lacking, smaller examples include a Togolese study that found moderate/severe anemia among U5s had declined 28% nine months after LLIN distribution (compared to before distribution).[151] A study in Liberia demonstrated that one year after distribution of Interceptor LLINs and conventional ITNs (treated with alpha-cypermethrin), significant decreases were seen in both population-wide *Plasmodium* spp. parasitemia (from 30% to 14% [p<.001]) and clinical malaria among children (from 8% to 2% [p<.001]). Although the authors did not report efficacy differences between the two types of bednets, the LLINs retained 78% of baseline insecticide, compared to only 7% among the conventional ITNs after one year of field use.[79] Although it is expected that U5 mortality and morbidity reductions with LLIN use will be similar to (or better than) that seen with conventional ITNs, little data currently exist, and further research is needed. The impact of the community effect has yet to be well evaluated in a large-scale LLIN trial.

Although there have been few direct comparisons of LLINs to conventional ITNs in field trials that have assessed morbidity and mortality, emerging data supports the hypothesis that LLINs are more wash-resistant and durable than conventional ITNs. In Western Kenya, significantly fewer PermaNet 1.0s lost their mosquito-killing effect than conventional ITNs treated with deltamethrin over a two-year follow-up, and other studies support the same conclusion.[80,87,95] Operational differences between LLIN and conventional ITN distribution programs generally favor LLINs, including the obviation of the need for insecticide retreatment every six months and the better durability of LLINs, although further research is needed. Though somewhat more expensive initially, LLINs are becoming more widely available and less expensive over time, and in many settings are now approaching conventional ITNs in cost. It seems likely that LLINs are demonstrably more cost-effective than conventional ITNs, and whether the logistical advantages of these nets indeed results in improved effectiveness with field use is another area in need of further research.

---

[151] D.J. Terlouw *et al.*, Impact of mass distribution of free long-lasting insecticidal nets on childhood malaria morbidity: the Togo National Integrated Child Health Campaign, *Malaria Journal*, 2010, **9**, 199.

ITN Efficacy: Conclusions

A 2004 Cochrane meta-analysis of ITN trials determined that 5.5 lives would be saved annually for every 1,000 U5s protected by ITNs (95%CI 3.4-7.7). ITNs also reduced the incidence of uncomplicated malaria in areas of stable malaria transmission by 50% compared to no nets, and by 39% compared to untreated bednets.[105] In areas of unstable malaria transmission, ITNs reduced the incidence of *P. falciparum* infection by 62% compared to no nets and by 43% compared to untreated bednets. ITNs also significantly reduced parasite prevalence, parasitemia, splenomegaly, and improved hemoglobin levels in U5s. This study estimated that in 2004, approximately 370,000 U5 deaths could be avoided if every U5 in sub-Saharan Africa was protected by an ITN.[105]

Although these data regarding the efficacy of ITNs are compelling, most evidence comes from trials in which ITNs were deployed under well-controlled conditions, leading to high coverage and use rates. Such conditions are not easily met in large-scale ITN distribution programs, and thus the real-world effectiveness of ITNs is likely less than the efficacy data presented above. As an example, the first ITN trial conducted in The Gambia achieved high coverage in the target population, and resulted in a childhood mortality reduction of 60%.[42,152] Later, an evaluation of a national Gambian bednet impregnation program which had a lower coverage rate reported a childhood mortality reduction of only 23%.[126,135] The gains seen near Kisumu, Kenya as a result of the Western Kenya ITN Trial were also somewhat reversed several years later, due in part to waning support for public health measures.[153] Large differences between efficacy and effectiveness such as this may be seen in many countries that lack the resources and experience necessary to properly implement large-scale ITN distribution.

Insecticide Resistance

The main biological threat to the efficacy of ITNs/LLINs is the development of insecticide resistance among anophelines.[154] Only six insecticides (all pyrethroids) have received full WHO approval for use in LLINs/ITNs.[64] Recently, two LLINs

---

[152]P.I. Alonso *et al.*, A malaria control trial using insecticide-treated bed nets and targeted chemoprophylaxis in a rural area of The Gambia, west Africa. 6. The impact of the interventions on mortality and morbidity from malaria, *Transactions of the Royal Society of Tropical Medicine and Hygiene*, 1993, **87**(Suppl 2), 37–44.

[153]M.J. Hamel *et al.*, A reversal in reductions of child mortality in Western Kenya, 2003–2009, *American Journal of Tropical Medicine and Hygiene*, 2011, **85**(4), 597–605.

[154]R.M. Oxborough *et al.*, Mosquitoes and bednets: testing the spatial positioning of insecticide on nets and the rationale behind combination insecticide treatments, *Annals of Tropical Medicine and Parasitology*, 2008, **102**(8), 717–27.

with non-pyrethroid based insecticides (PermaNet 3.0 and Olyset Plus) received interim WHO approval.[92] Although WHO has approved twelve insecticides for IRS, these belong to just four chemical classes. Because the mechanism of action for all four is similar, the development of resistance is a concern.[155]

Pyrethroid resistance was first detected in African anophelines in 1993, and the gene that confers knockdown resistance to pyrethroids (kdr) has now been described. This mutation is already present in *Anopheles gambiae* in many areas of West Africa[156,157] and has also been documented in parts of East Africa.[158] Although initially a minor concern, kdr is now a significant threat to the long-term effectiveness of ITNs.[159,160]

A 2008 study of an LLIN distribution program in Niger revealed a rapid increase in the frequency of the kdr-w mutation among *An. gambiae* after an LLIN distribution campaign in 2005, from 0.5% in 2005 to 7.0% by 2007.[161] A recent experimental hut trial in Benin demonstrated that the mortality of *An. gambiae* exposed to ITNs in areas without suspected pyrethroid resistance was 98%, while in areas of known resistance the mortality rate was only 30%.[159] The authors concluded that pyrethroid resistance in *An. gambiae* could threaten the future effectiveness of ITNs and IRS in Benin.

The kdr mutation is one of two major resistance mechanisms. A second stems from over-expression of several anopheline enzymes that metabolize pyrethroids. In southern Africa, the emergence of *An. funestus* with pyrethroid resistance was associated with upregulated cytochrome P450 activity and was possibly responsible for the increase in malaria burden in KwaZulu-Natal (South Africa) between

---

[155]J. Hemingway *et al.*, The molecular basis of insecticide resistance in mosquitoes, *Insect Biochemistry and Molecular Biology*, 2004, **34**(7), 653–65.

[156]J. Pinto *et al.*, Co-occurrence of East and West African kdr mutations suggests high levels of resistance to pyrethroid insecticides in *Anopheles gambiae* from Libreville, Gabon, *Medical and Veterinary Entomology*, 2006, **20**(1), 27–32.

[157]J. Etang *et al.*, First report of knockdown mutations in the malaria vector *Anopheles gambiae* from Cameroon, *American Journal of Tropical Medicine and Hygiene*, 2006, **74**(5), 795–7.

[158]J.M. Vulule *et al.*, Reduced susceptibility of *Anopheles gambiae* to permethrin associated with the use of permethrin-impregnated bednets and curtains in Kenya, *Medical and Veterinary Entomology*, 1994, **8**(1), 71–5.

[159]R. N'Guessan *et al.*, Reduced efficacy of insecticide-treated nets and indoor residual spraying for malaria control in pyrethroid resistance area, Benin, *Emerging Infectious Disease*, 2007, **13**(2), 199–206.

[160]B.L. Sharp *et al.*, Malaria vector control by indoor residual insecticide spraying on the tropical island of Bioko, Equatorial Guinea, *Malaria Journal*, 2007, **6**, 52.

[161]C. Czeher *et al.*, Evidence of increasing Leu-Phe knockdown resistance mutation in *Anopheles gambiae* from Niger following a nationwide long-lasting insecticide-treated nets implementation, *Malaria Journal*, 2008, **7**, 189.

1995 and 1999.[162] *An. funestus*, a highly anthropophilic vector, re-emerged after previously disappearing from the area when IRS was introduced. This mechanism of resistance has also been observed in *An. gambiae* populations in Cameroon, Kenya, Benin, Ghana and South Africa.[163–165]

Though alarming, these studies occurred mostly in areas where pyrethroids were used not only for ITNs, but also for IRS and agriculture, resulting in higher selection pressure. Agricultural use of pyrethroids, primarily in cotton-growing areas, has contributed to resistance in *An. gambiae* in Cote d'Ivoire, Benin, and Burkina Faso.[166–168]

Some evidence suggests that pyrethroid-treated bednets maintain effectiveness even after extensive use in a defined geographic area. In Tanzania, where pyrethroid-treated bednets have been used for up to 17 years, *Anopheles spp.* mortality was >90% after standard WHO susceptibility tests in almost all areas of the country.[169] Some evidence indicates that pyrethroid-treated bednets can still be effective against kdr homozygous mosquitoes.[170] In an experimental hut trial, pyrethroid-treated ITNs still killed >95% of kdr homozygous anophelines from Burkina Faso, and Côte d'Ivoire.[63] One possible explanation is that kdr reduces the irritant effect of pyrethroids, resulting in mosquitoes resting for longer periods on pyrethroid-treated ITNs, increasing exposure to the insecticide. Similar results have been

[162.] K. Hargreaves *et al.*, *Anopheles funestus* resistant to pyrethroid insecticides in South Africa, *Medical and Veterinary Entomology*, 2000, **14**(2), 181–9.

[163] J.M. Vulule *et al.*, Elevated oxidase and esterase levels associated with permethrin tolerance in *Anopheles gambiae* from Kenyan villages using permethrin-impregnated nets, *Medical and Veterinary Entomology*, 1999, **13**(3), 239–44.

[164] J. Etang *et al.*, Reduced bio-efficacy of permethrin EC impregnated bednets against an *Anopheles gambiae* strain with oxidase-based pyrethroid tolerance, *Malaria Journal*, 2004, **3**, 46.

[165] V. Corbel *et al.*, Field efficacy of a new mosaic long-lasting mosquito net (PermaNet 3.0) against pyrethroid-resistant malaria vectors: a multi centre study in Western and Central Africa, *Malaria Journal*, 2010, **9**, 113.

[166] M. Akogbeto and S. Yakoubou, Resistance of malaria vectors to pyrethrins used for impregnating mosquito nets in Benin, West Africa, *Bulletin de la Société de pathologie exotique*, 1999, **92**(2), 123–30.

[167] F. Chandre *et al.*, Status of pyrethroid resistance in *Anopheles gambiae* sensu lato, *Bulletin of the World Health Organisation*, 1999, **77**(3), 203–34.

[168] A. Diabate *et al.*, The role of agricultural use of insecticides in resistance to pyrethroids in *Anopheles gambiae* s.l. in Burkina Faso, *American Journal of Tropical Medicine and Hygeine*, 2002, **67**(6), 617–22.

[169] M.A. Kulkarni *et al.*, Efficacy of pyrethroid-treated nets against malaria vectors and nuisance-biting mosquitoes in Tanzania in areas with long-term insecticide-treated net use, *Tropical Medicine and International Health*, 2007, **12**(9), 1061–73.

[170] G. Munhenga *et al.*, Pyrethroid resistance in the major malaria vector *Anopheles arabiensis* from Gwave, a malaria-endemic area in Zimbabwe, *Malaria Journal*, 2008, **7**, 247.

found in other trials.[69,171] Conversely, while few studies have documented that higher insecticide resistance rates have resulted in increased malaria morbidity or mortality, a recent study in Senegal suggested that this may now be occurring. There, 2–3 years after PermaNet 2.0 deployment in a village, kdr frequency among *An. gambiae* increased from 8% to 48%. Clinical malaria episodes had initially decreased significantly (from pre-distribution baseline) just after LLIN deployment, but re-increased nearly back to baseline after pyrethroid resistance became more widespread.[134]

To improve monitoring capability, the WHO/Tropical Disease Research network on insecticide resistance in African malaria vectors was established in 2008. Areas where large-scale insecticide-based control programs are operational but without resistance data were prioritized for early surveillance activities. Three of the five countries surveyed in the first year of the program (Burkina Faso, Chad, and Sudan) contained high frequencies of resistant *An. gambiae* and the prevalence of resistance has increased in all three countries compared to earlier data.[172,173] In Chad, for example, *An. gambiae* mortality after standardized exposure to permethrin decreased from 60% to 43% between 2006 and 2008, and from 73% to 31% for deltamethrin.

In response to increasing pyrethroid resistance, bednet manufacturers have developed "mosaic" LLINs. One example (PermaNet 3.0) employs a pyrethroid (deltamethrin) on the net's sides and deltamethrin combined with a synergistic, non-pyrethroid insecticide (piperonyl butoxide; PBO) on the net's roof. The more toxic non-pyrethroid insecticide is thus farther from the sleeper, while sides are impregnated with only the less toxic pyrethroid. For this strategy to be successful, anophelines must have at least the same propensity to land on the top of the ITN as on the sides. This was tested in Northern Tanzania where *An. arabiensis* mortality was almost identical in bednets treated with a pyrethroid on the top only, sides only, and all surfaces, suggesting that *An. arabiensis* contacts the top and sides of an ITN equally during host-seeking behavior.[154] This type of ITN is also more effective against culicines, which are more resistant to pyrethroids than anophelines. By reducing other mosquitoes such as these, ITNs could increase bednet compliance.[174]

[171] J. Etang *et al.*, Insecticide susceptibility status of *Anopheles gambiae* s.l. (Diptera: Culicidae) in the Republic of Cameroon, *Journal of Medical Entomology*, 2003, **40**(4), 491–7.

[172] H. Ranson *et al.*, Insecticide resistance in *Anopheles gambiae*: data from the first year of a multi-country study highlight the extent of the problem, *Malaria Journal*, 2009, **8**(1), 299.

[173] WHO, Report of the Informal WHO Consultation: Test procedures for insecticide resistance monitoring in malaria vectors, bio-efficacy and presistence of insecticide on treated surfaces, WHO, 1998, 3–28: Geneva, Switzerland.

[174] P. Guillet *et al.*, Combined pyrethroid and carbamate 'two-in-one' treated mosquito nets: field efficacy against pyrethroid-resistant *Anopheles gambiae* and *Culex quinquefasciatus*, *Medical and Veterinary Entomology*, 2001, **15**(1), 105–12.

PBO enhances the effects of deltamethrin by inhibiting anopheline enzymes such as cytochrome P450.[175] A recent study compared the efficacy of PermaNet 3.0 to deltamethrin-only treated ITNs in Burkina Faso, at a site where the kdr mutation was present in >80% of *An. gambiae*. In this area, PermaNet 3.0 was more effective at inhibiting feeding and resulted in higher mosquito mortality than the pyrethroid-only LLINs, suggesting that the combination of insecticides on this LLIN may be successful even against resistant vectors.[165] However, it was unclear if this improved efficacy against resistant vectors was due to the presence of PBO or the higher deltamethrin content in PermaNet 3.0. Many mosquitoes still survived exposure to the mosaic net in high-resistance areas. Whether PermaNet 3.0 is a viable long-term strategy against pyrethroid-resistant mosquitoes remains to be seen, and WHOPES has not yet endorsed the manufacturer's assertion that PermaNet 3.0 is effective against resistant vectors.[94,100]

Although still an emerging problem, pyrethroid-resistant anophelines are a major threat to the effectiveness of ITN programs for controlling malaria. Further research is needed, including an examination of different insecticide classes for IRS and ITN/LLINs in locations where both control measures are being used, better monitoring for insecticide resistance in areas with these programs, and development of new insecticides/insecticide combinations on ITNs.

Cost-effectiveness of ITNs/LLINs

Although generally less expensive than LLINs, conventional ITNs require retreatment every six months, an expensive and logistically challenging endeavor. A 2008 analysis found that LLINs were significantly more cost-effective over the life of the bednet than either conventionally treated ITNs or IRS.[84] Assuming that LLINs are effective for three years and used properly, an analysis of the Togo Integrated Campaign showed that the annual cost per death avoided was $773 for LLINs and $1,174 for ITNs (Table 4).[176]

Others have found that the cost per life saved for LLINs is less than half that for conventional ITNs.[53] In high-transmission areas, LLIN programs are less expensive than IRS programs. The annual cost per LLIN averages $2.10 (range $1.48–2.64), or $1.05 per person protected per year.[76]

---

[175]G. Bingham *et al.*, Temporal synergism by microencapsulation of piperonyl butoxide and alpha-cypermethrin overcomes insecticide resistance in crop pests, *Pest Management Science*, 2007, **63**(3), 276–81.

[176]J.O. Yukich, T. Fabrizio and C. Lengeler, Operations, Costs and Cost-Effectiveness of Five Insecticide-Treated Net Programs (Eritrea, Malawi, Tanzania, Togo, Senegal) and Two Indoor Residual Spraying Programs (Kwa-Zulu-Natal, Mozambique), Swiss Tropical Institute, 2007, 112–23: Basel.

Although both IRS and ITNs are highly effective (and similar in their impact) against malaria, free ITN distribution campaigns appear to be more cost-effective than IRS in low income, highly malaria-endemic settings.[177,178] One model supporting this view found that in a low-income country, the cost per disability-adjusted life year saved was $4–10 for an ITN, $19 for an ITN plus annual insecticide retreatments, and $32–58 for twice-annual IRS.[178,179]

A comparison of five ITN and two IRS programs determined that ITNs are more cost-effective than IRS in highly malaria-endemic settings, especially if high community ITN coverage can be achieved. The cost per treated net-year of protection ranged from $1.21 in Eritrea to $6.05 in Senegal and the cost per death averted ranged from $438–2,199. IRS costs were higher: $21.63–23.90 per person-year of protection and $3,933–4,357 per death avoided.[176,177] Modeling has also suggested that ITNs are the most effective single option for malaria prevention.[180]

However, ITNs/LLINs alone are likely inadequate to eliminate malaria; a multi-pronged approach (including IRS and effective case management) is necessary.[6,180,181] One study which demonstrated the benefits of a multi-pronged approach found that IRS combined with LLINs reduced the risk of malaria infection more effectively in Equatorial Guinea (OR = 0.71, 95%CI 0.59–0.86) and Mozambique (OR = 0.63, 95%CI 0.50–0.79) than IRS alone.[182]

Overall, while ITNs/LLINs and IRS are both effective for malaria control, ITNs/LLINs appear to be more cost-effective.[183] The Roll Back Malaria partnership concluded that the choose between IRS and ITNs in a given area should be determined by availability of local resources, operational capability, and potential for sustained coverage. However, a consensus seems to be emerging that LLINs are the most cost-effective vector-based approach for malaria control in

---

[177] J.O. Yukich *et al.*, Costs and consequences of large-scale vector control for malaria, *Malaria Journal*, 2008, **7**, 258.

[178] C.A. Goodman, P.G. Coleman and A.J. Mills, Cost-effectiveness of malaria control in sub-Saharan Africa, *Lancet*, 1999, **354**(9176), 378–85.

[179] C.A. Goodman *et al.*, Comparison of the cost and cost-effectiveness of insecticide-treated bednets and residual house-spraying in KwaZulu-Natal, South Africa, *Tropical Medicine and International Health*, 2001, **6**(4), 280–95.

[180] N. Chitnis *et al.*, Comparing the effectiveness of malaria vector-control interventions through a mathematical model, *American Journal of Tropical Medicine and Hygiene*, 2010, **83**(2), 230–40.

[181] J.T. Griffin *et al.*, Reducing *Plasmodium falciparum* malaria transmission in Africa: a model-based evaluation of intervention strategies, *Public Library of Science Medicine*, 2010, **7**(8), e1000324.

[182] I. Kleinschmidt *et al.*, Combining indoor residual spraying and insecticide-treated net interventions, *American Journal of Tropical Medicine and Hygiene*, 2009, **81**(3), 519–24.

[183] WHO, RBM, Scaling up Insecticide-treated Netting Programmes in Africa, 2005, 4–23: Geneva, Switzerland.

Table 4: Cost-effectiveness of the Togo integrated campaign.

	Conventional ITNs	**LLINs**
Deaths averted	2,487	7,462
DALYs averted	82,083	246,250
Annual cost per death averted	$1,174	$773
Annual cost per DALY averted	$36	$23

DALY: Disability-adjusted life year
Adapted from (Yukich *et al.*, 2007)[176]

areas of high malaria transmission. LLINs seem clearly superior in areas with a long season of (or perennial) malaria transmission (requiring >1 annual IRS cycle), or in areas where IRS cannot be used (e.g., forest malaria or among nomadic populations).[184] Still, IRS does reduce the vector population quickly and may be preferred in certain situations, such as containing malaria outbreaks, controlling malaria in complex emergencies, areas of intense transmission (to rapidly and substantially reduce malaria), epidemic-prone areas, foci with low seasonal transmission or seasonal transmission peaks, and areas where LLINs may be ineffective due to pyrethroid resistance.[185]

ITN/LLIN Policy, Distribution and Use

ITN/LLIN distribution

Although there is little debate regarding the efficacy of ITNs/LLINs for preventing malaria, controversies remain regarding the best means to distribute them. WHO now recommends that malaria/vector-control programs distribute only LLINs, via free or highly subsidized means, such that the entire population at-risk for malaria is protected. While this is a laudable goal, these recommendations do not address the sustainability of such programs, particularly in the resource-limited settings in which malaria is most commonly endemic. Where resources are limited and insufficient ITNs/LLINs are present to cover entire populations, an open question remains whether it is better to initially cover U5s and PW widely, or to focus initially on full population coverage in the highest-risk areas. Alternatively, attempts at wider distribution using cost-recovery mechanisms

---

[184]WHO, Global Malaria Programme, Malaria: Global Fund Proposal Development (Round 11), WHO, 1–35: Geneva, Switzerland.
[185]A. Kilian *et al.*, How many mosquito nets are needed to achieve universal coverage? Recommendations for the quantification and allocation of long-lasting insecticidal nets for mass campaigns, *Malaria Journal*, 2010, **9**, 330.

would likely allow expansion of the geographic regions covered, at the risk of decreasing compliance with the program compared to free ITN distribution. While the balance of current recommendations and evidence favors high overall coverage as a goal (in large part because of the ITN community effect), this approach has not been robustly compared to wider coverage schemes that initially target the vulnerable population followed by subsequent scale-up. One group estimates that one LLIN is needed for every 1.6 people to achieve universal coverage.[185] WHO currently recommends allocating one LLIN for every 1.8–2.0 people in a community.[184]

The primary dilemma related to the distribution and use of ITNs over the past 15 years has stemmed from the difficulty inherent to the competing demands between equity and sustainability of ITN/LLIN distribution programs and achieving high coverage and use rates. Most populations at-risk for malaria live in rural, impoverished communities, with limited means to pay for ITNs/LLINs. In addition, health infrastructure in most of Africa is poorly organized and funded, and faces a number of pressing public health problems in addition to malaria.

Distribution systems

Mass ITN/LLIN distribution programs face unique logistical challenges because of the relative bulk and weight of ITNs/LLINs compared to other large-scale health campaigns such as vaccination or mass drug administration; this engenders significant storage, transport, and other logistical concerns for ITN campaigns that mass drug administration and vaccination campaigns do not face. ITNs can be distributed at central locations, and such programs are logistically easier to perform than house-to-house campaigns but generally result in lower ITN uptake. The debate over distribution mechanisms for ITNs/LLINs centers largely over whether they are public or private goods, and the respective roles of the public and private sector in their delivery.[186,187] Roll Back Malaria has proposed a two-pronged approach: targeted and sustained subsidies for those at greatest risk, coupled with the development of the commercial sector.[183]

One means to achieve successful and targeted distribution is to link ITN/LLIN campaigns to other established programs such as mass drug administration and immunization campaigns, which already have the human and logistical resources in place for large-scale distribution. This strategy can increase coverage and

---

[186] C. Curtis *et al.*, Scaling-up coverage with insecticide-treated nets against malaria in Africa: who should pay?, *Lancet Infectious Disease*, 2003, **3**(5), 304–7.

[187] J. Lines *et al.*, Scaling-up and sustaining insecticide-treated net coverage, *Lancet Infectious Disease*, 2003, **3**(8), 465–6

decrease costs.[188,189] Distribution of ITNs through programs that are integrated with other mass public health campaigns may be the way forward.

Several programs which have integrated ITN/LLIN distribution with other mass public health campaigns have been successful in sub-Saharan Africa. In 2003, ITN distribution integrated with measles vaccination, vitamin A, and mebendazole distribution in Zambia resulted in >80% coverage for all interventions, with 89,000 U5s participating within a week.[190] In Togo (2004), integrated ITN distribution, measles and polio vaccination, plus albendazole administration resulted in 920,000 ITNs distributed and increased overall household ITN possession from 6% to 62%; 98% of households with an U5 owned an ITN after this campaign.[190] Malawi had success beginning in 2002–04 by integrating ITN distribution with antenatal care (ANC), where the number of ITNs distributed increased from 750,000 in 2002 to 3,000,000 in 2004, and household ITN ownership increasing from 5% in 2000 to 43% in 2004.[190] The first program which integrated ITN distribution with a lymphatic filariasis/onchocerciasis mass drug administration (MDA) campaign was also successful, distributing nearly 40,000 ITNs in less than six months in 2004 in Central Nigeria. The program increased the number of households owning an ITN from 9% to 80% and increased U5 ITN use from <5% to 37% while also benefitting the existing MDA program.[191] In Tanzania, integrating LLIN distribution with existing measles immunization programs increased ITN/LLIN ownership nationally from 46% to 63% and U5 ITN/LLIN usage from 29% to 64% from 2009 to 2010.[189] A similar program in Niger increased LLIN ownership from 6% to 65% by integrating LLIN distribution with a polio vaccination campaign.[192]

Public-based free delivery systems have been responsible for much of the recent increase in ITN coverage, and the poorest sectors of society are most effectively

---

[188] D.H. Molyneux and V.M. Nantulya, Linking disease control programmes in rural Africa: a pro-poor strategy to reach Abuja targets and millennium development goals, *British Medical Journal*, 2004, **328**(7448), 1129–32.

[189] K. Bonner *et al.*, Design, implementation and evaluation of a national campaign to distribute nine million free LLINs to children under five years of age in Tanzania, *Malaria Journal*, 2011, **10**(1), 73.

[190] WHO, Global Malaria Programme, World Malaria Report 2005, WHO, 2005, 22–31: Geneva, Switzerland.

[191] B.G. Blackburn *et al.*, Successful integration of insecticide-treated bed net distribution with mass drug administration in Central Nigeria, *American Journal of Tropical Medicine and Hygeine*, 2006, **75**(4), 650–5.

[192] J. Thwing *et al.*, Insecticide-treated net ownership and usage in Niger after a nationwide integrated campaign, *Tropical Medicine and International Health*, 2008, **13**(6), 827–34.

targeted by free, public delivery.[6,186,193,194] The community effect is also best achieved with mass, free ITN/LLIN distribution. When high coverage is achieved, ITNs/LLINs may be viewed as public goods, protecting both users and non-users from malaria. A drawback to this strategy involves sustainability, as poor countries lack the resources to purchase and distribute large numbers of free ITNs/LLINs, and instead must rely on donors.

In Uganda, LLINs are distributed through two public-sector channels: targeted delivery campaigns or routine antenatal care services. The cost per LLIN used was $2.31 for the antenatal clinics and $1.10 through LLIN delivery campaigns. Delivery through ANCs was more expensive because this strategy took longer, and required supervision, tracking, and storage of LLIN supplies over longer periods of time. Both strategies achieved high coverage.[195]

In contrast, distribution through the private sector is more sustainable, as funding from governments or non-governmental organizations (NGOs) is not required. Although private sector ITN/LLIN delivery may at first appear to be the least equitable system, this remains controversial.[186] One group estimated that in 2005, most of the children in Africa protected by bednets in the early 2000s used untreated bednets. Despite the fact that untreated bednets were usually purchased through the private sector, untreated bednet coverage was as equitable as common free public health measures such as EPI (the Expanded Programme on Immunization). The same study found that ITNs (presumably distributed by public health programs) were concentrated mostly in the least-poor households. Taken together, these results suggest that the public health value of the commercial bednet market had been under-utilized, and may have done more for equitable bednet distribution than free public health ITN distribution programs had to that point. This contradicted other studies which showed that free, public ITN/LLIN distribution achieved the highest coverage among vulnerable, low-income groups, although this study was based on data obtained before completion of the major ITN/LLIN distribution campaigns of recent years.[196]

---

[193] M. De Allegri *et al.*, Comparative cost analysis of insecticide-treated net delivery strategies: sales supported by social marketing and free distribution through antenatal care, *Health Policy Plan*, 2010, **25**(1), 28–38.

[194] A.M. Noor *et al.*, Increasing coverage and decreasing inequity in insecticide-treated bed net use among rural Kenyan children, *Public Library of Science Medicine*, 2007, **4**(8), e255.

[195] J.H. Kolaczinski *et al.*, Costs and effects of two public sector delivery channels for long-lasting insecticidal nets in Uganda, *Malaria Journal*, 2010, **9**, 102.

[196] J. Webster *et al.*, Which delivery systems reach the poor? A review of equity of coverage of ever-treated nets, never-treated nets, and immunisation to reduce child mortality in Africa, *Lancet Infectious Disease*, 2005, **5**(11), 709–17.

Although the private sector approach is aided by reduction of taxes/tariffs on nets, netting materials and insecticides, less than half of African counties have done this.[197] Following the reduction or removal of tariffs, private sector ITN/LLIN distribution increased in Uganda, Tanzania, and Zambia.[183,198]

Some distribution strategies combine public and private approaches. A commonly cited example is the voucher scheme, where subsidized ITNs/LLINs are delivered through the public sector, and sold through the private sector. This allows targeting of subsidies in the public sector, while allowing the private sector to benefit from the sale. In many African countries, the delivery of partially subsidized ITNs through routine health facilities and voucher schemes is supported by NGOs.[198–201] However, a comparative cost analysis of ITN distribution in Burkina Faso through a social marketing voucher scheme and free distribution through clinics found that free distribution was less expensive to implement than social marketing ($7.21 vs. $8.08 per ITN distributed) [1943]. A related study found that higher coverage was achieved in villages that received free ITNs through antenatal clinics (35% vs. 23%; p < 0.001) than a group that was exposed to social marketing but did not receive free ITNs.[200]

Considerable overlap exists between public and private sector delivery options. It is even possible that public sector ITN/LLIN delivery undermines the private sector by flooding the market with free ITNs/LLINs. One recent study found that the highest household ITN ownership (63%) was achieved through public-free delivery, (e.g., in conjunction with antenatal clinics, child health weeks, or vaccination campaigns), while use by PW and U5s (67%) was highest through private-unsubsidized delivery (e.g., via employer-based systems, non-profit organizations, and the retail sector).[201,202]

Overall, free LLIN distribution seems to achieve the best coverage and is the only feasible means to achieve high coverage rates in impoverished areas.

[197] M. Alilio *et al.*, Broken promise? Taxes and tariffs on insecticide treated mosquito nets, *American Journal of Tropical Medicine and Hygiene*, 2007, **77**(6 Suppl), 227–31.

[198] D.G. Wacira *et al.*, Delivery of insecticide-treated net services through employer and community-based approaches in Kenya, *Tropical Medicine and International Health*, 2007, **12**(1), 140–9.

[199] J. Omona, Social marketing and the fight against malaria in Africa: population services international (PSI) and insecticide treated nets (ITNs), *East African Journal of Public Health*, 2009, **6**(3), 317–25.

[200] O. Muller *et al.*, Distribution systems of insecticide-treated bed nets for malaria control in rural Burkina Faso: cluster-randomized controlled trial, *Public Library of Science One*, 2008, **3**(9), e3182.

[201] J. Webster *et al.*, Delivery systems for insecticide treated and untreated mosquito nets in Africa: categorization and outcomes achieved, *Health Policy Plan*, 2007, **22**(5), 277–93.

[202] J. Kolaczinski and K. Hanson, Costing the distribution of insecticide-treated nets: a review of cost and cost-effectiveness studies to provide guidance on standardization of costing methodology, *Malaria Journal*, 2006, **5**, 37.

Integrating with other public health programs may be the way forward, but continued international funding is necessary to continue the recent gains. Achieving high community-wide coverage in the most highly malaria-endemic areas seems the best initial approach, given that the impact of the community effect is best achieved in this setting. However, different strategies offer unique advantages and disadvantages that depend on the socioeconomic and entomologic setting. There is a need for standardization of costing methodologies and coverage outcomes so that different delivery systems can be empirically compared.

Factors affecting ITN compliance

Even in settings where ITNs are distributed widely and ownership or accessibility is not a problem, ITN use by households that own them (compliance) is an important consideration for distribution programs. In the setting of randomized controlled trials, ITN use increases initially, but decreases over time, raising the concern that under the real-world conditions of mass campaigns, ITN/LLIN use will be lower than under study conditions. Such concern has been mitigated somewhat by recent household surveys that demonstrate 80% ITN use across many countries years following mass ITN/LLIN distributions.[6,203,204]

A range of environmental, social, and economic factors influence ITN/LLIN adherence.[205] These include age, gender, temperature/season, knowledge of malaria/transmission patterns, socio-economic status, and perceived value of ITNs/LLINs. Studies have shown varying results regarding whether an individual factor negatively or positively affects ITN/LLIN use, depending on the specific setting. Hotter temperatures seem to consistently influence adherence negatively, and increased mosquito density results in higher adherence.[57,205–208] Studies examin-

[203] J.L. Vanden Eng *et al.*, Assessing bed net use and non-use after long-lasting insecticidal net distribution: a simple framework to guide programmatic strategies, *Malaria Journal*, 2010, **9**, 133.

[204] T.P. Eisele *et al.*, Assessment of insecticide-treated bednet use among children and pregnant women across 15 countries using standardized national surveys, *American Journal of Tropical Medicine and Hygiene*, 2009, **80**(2), 209–14.

[205] J.A. Alaii *et al.*, Factors affecting use of permethrin-treated bed nets during a randomized controlled trial in western Kenya, *American Journal of Tropical Medicine and Hygiene*, 2003, **68**(4 Suppl), 137–41.

[206] J. Pulford *et al.*, Reported reasons for not using a mosquito net when one is available: a review of the published literature, *Malaria Journal*, 2011, **10**, 83.

[207] F.N. Binka and P. Adongo, Acceptability and use of insecticide impregnated bednets in northern Ghana, *Tropical Medicine and International Health*, 1997, **2**(5), 499–507.

[208] M. Gyapong *et al.*, Introducing insecticide impregnated bednets in an area of low bednet usage: an exploratory study in north-east Ghana, *Tropical Medicine and International Health*, 1996, **1**(3), 328–33.

ing the impact of whether an ITN was purchased or received for free on adherence have shown that high ITN compliance can be seen when ITNs are received for free (refuting the previously held belief that such ITNs would be less valued and used less).[194,209,210] Other studies have shown that offering financial incentives to increase ITN use are effective.[211]

In the Western Kenya ITN Trial, approximately 30% of ITNs went unused. U5s were less likely to use ITNs than older individuals, and ITN use was more likely during cooler weather. Mosquito numbers, relative wealth, household size, and educational level had no effect on compliance. Excessive heat was often cited as a reason for non-use, while the most important reason for noncompliance was disruption of sleeping arrangements. It seems clear that temperature and seasonality play a major role in compliance, as multiple studies have demonstrated that bednet use declines during the hot season in many locales.[192,205] Other studies (e.g., in Ethiopia) have seemingly contradicted these, showing that higher educational attainment and higher wealth indices are positively correlated with ITN/LLIN use. Owning ITNs/LLINs that were older or more damaged was associated with lower bednet use rates in that location, suggesting that upkeep programs may have an important impact on both ITN efficacy and compliance.[212,213]

Recent surveys suggest a changing pattern of gender and age-based adherence. Analyses of nine large-scale household surveys in 2000–2004 revealed that among ITN/LLIN owners in six African countries, reproductive-age women and U5s were the most likely household members to use bednets, and children aged 5–14 and adult males were the least likely. In Zambia, the proportion of pregnant women who used ITNs increased from 18% in 2000 to 51% 2004.[214] These

[209] H. Guyatt and S. Ochola, Use of bednets given free to pregnant women in Kenya, *Lancet*, 2003, **362**(9395), 1549–50.

[210] A.M. Noor *et al.*, Insecticide-treated net coverage in Africa: mapping progress in 2000–07, *Lancet*, 2009, **373**(9657), 58–67.

[211] P.J. Krezanoski, A.B. Comfort and D.H. Hamer, Effect of incentives on insecticide-treated bed net use in sub-Saharan Africa: a cluster randomized trial in Madagascar, *Malaria Journal*, 2010, **9**, 186.

[212] M. Belay and W. Deressa, Use of insecticide treated nets by pregnant women and associated factors in a pre-dominantly rural population in northern Ethiopia, *Tropical Medicine and International Health*, 2008, **13**(10), 1303–13.

[213] J.M. Ngondi *et al.*, Which nets are being used: factors associated with mosquito net use in Amhara, Oromia and Southern Nations, Nationalities and Peoples' Regions of Ethiopia, *Malaria Journal*, 2011, **10**, 92.

[214] C.A. Baume and M.C. Marin, Intra-household mosquito net use in Ethiopia, Ghana, Mali, Nigeria, Senegal, and Zambia: are nets being used? Who in the household uses them?, *American Journal of Tropical Medicine and Hygiene*, 2007, **77**(5), 963–71.

contrast with past studies which suggested that in households owning ITNs, adult males used bednets at the expense of U5s and PWs.[205,215,216]

Large-scale ITN/LLIN distribution directly to PW and mothers with children through antenatal clinics and the EPI program may explain the recent rise in ITN/ LLIN use among women and children. Another factor is the linkage of malaria control to ITN/LLIN education programs, which provides information regarding the susceptibility of pregnant women to severe malaria and mitigation of fears about possible adverse effects of insecticides. Zambia made remarkable strides in this area, with only 7% of pregnant women expressing concern about insecticides in 2004, compared to 27% in 2000.[217]

ITN distribution campaigns often contain an educational component designed to teach the local population about the means of malaria transmission, the consequences of malaria, and the effectiveness of ITNs in preventing malaria. These informational campaigns are an essential component of any ITN distribution program, with the goal of increasing adherence through better knowledge, attitudes, and practices. Combining such education with ITN distribution significantly increases usage compared to mass distribution campaigns with no educational component.[140,194,218]

Recent Progress and Conclusions

In the past decade, substantial progress has been made toward universal access to ITNs/LLINs for all persons at risk for malaria. By 2009, the malaria control policy of 65 countries included the WHO recommendation of LLIN provision to all persons at risk for malaria. Eighty-three countries now distribute LLINs free of charge. Global funding for malaria control increased from US $0.3 billion in 2003 to US $1.8 billion in 2010. Although >$6 billion annually may be necessary to successfully control malaria, this dramatic increase in funding has resulted in the scale-up of malaria control measures in many endemic countries with a consequent improvement in malaria indices.[6]

[215]J. Okrah *et al.*, Community factors associated with malaria prevention by mosquito nets: an exploratory study in rural Burkina Faso, *Tropical Medicine and International Health*, 2002, **7**(3), 240–8.

[216]B.A. Okech *et al.*, Use of integrated malaria management reduces malaria in Kenya, *Public Library of Science One*, 2008, **3**(12), e4050.

[217]U.S. Agency for International Development, NetMark, NetMark 2004 survey on insecticide-treated nets (ITNs) in Zambia, 2004. 39–50: Washington, D.C., USA.

[218]M. Widmar *et al.*, Determining and addressing obstacles to the effective use of long-lasting insecticide-impregnated nets in rural Tanzania, *Malaria Journal*, 2009, **8**, 315.

While some countries still struggle with ITN access, many successes are emerging. A 2007 report estimated that 17 million ITNs were deployed at that time.[219] While household surveys for 27 malaria-endemic countries between 2003 and 2009 reported only 17% household ITN ownership, more recent data are encouraging. Between 2008 and 2010, 289 million ITNs were delivered to sub-Saharan Africa (nearly all of which were LLINs), with household LLIN owner-ship now estimated at 53%.[220] While short of the coverage goals set by the international community, approximately 35% of U5s are now sleeping under ITNs, a substantial increase from the estimate of 3% just a few years ago.[6,210] An additional 35 million LLINs were scheduled for delivery before the end of 2010.[6] While it is difficult to separate the impact of ITN/LLIN distribution from other malaria control measures, modeling suggests that ITN/LLIN distribution has played a significant role in reducing malaria on a regional and global scale.[180] Twelve countries with successful ITN distribution programs experienced reduc-tions of >50% in either confirmed malaria cases or malaria admissions and deaths.[3] Of 56 malaria-endemic countries outside Africa, 32 achieved >50% reduction in the number of malaria cases between 2000 and 2009, while down-ward trends were seen in eight others countries.[3] Elimination of malaria was certified in three countries (Armenia, Morocco and Turkmenistan) between 2009 and 2011.[6,220]

Encouragingly, the estimated number of malaria cases globally dropped from 244 million in 2005 to 219 million in 2010, with estimated malaria deaths also dropping from 985,000 in 2000 to 660,000 in 2010.[220] From 2001–2010, scaling up of malaria prevention efforts, including LLINs, has saved the lives of nearly 1.1 million people globally.[220]

Despite these successes, challenges remain. In 2009, the malaria burden increased in three African countries where substantial progress had been seen previously (Rwanda, Sao Tome and Principe, and Zambia). Such increases highlight the fragility of malaria control and the need to maintain programs consistently. Replacement of LLINs (designed to last three years) that have been distributed in the above time frame will be necessary soon, and failure to do so could lead to a resurgence of malaria. Better surveillance systems are also needed, as many countries are unable to accurately monitor disease trends. Another challenge is the emerging resistance of some anophelines to the pyrethroid-based insecticides used in ITN/LLINs and some IRS programs.

---

[219] J.M. Miller *et al.*, Estimating the number of insecticide-treated nets required by African house-holds to reach continent-wide malaria coverage targets, *Journal of the American Medical Association*, 2007, **297**(20), 2241–50.
[220] WHO, Global Malaria Programme, World Malaria Report 2012, 2012, 1–62: Geneva Switerland.

Finally, finding for malaria control (and correspondingly, the number of ITNS procured) levelled off in 2011–2012, after previously being on an upward trend for a decade. Additionally, although hopefully not a sign of a larger trend, the number of malaria cases and deaths globally have also plateaved over the same time period, after dropping sharply for most of the decade prior to that.

Still, for the first time in decades, malaria control and elimination is benefitting from the support of the world community. Advocacy, awareness, and funding for malaria control are at their highest levels in recent memory, with most malaria indicators now revealing substantial progress. LLINs are a key component of a new global strategy to control and possibly eradicate malaria. Malaria eradication is a concept that was first embraced during the Global Malaria Eradication Program, launched in 1955 before being abandoned 15 years later. For the first time since, the world community is beginning to believe again that malaria eradication might be possible, especially given the recent success of some malaria control programs. However, a more realistic assessment suggests that eradication may not be possible for the immediate future. As with any elimination or eradication program, the incremental cost in going from a low-endemic setting to elimination is a major obstacle. Even for a small island like Zanzibar, on which malaria prevalence recently decreased to <2%, it would take 25 years before elimination would be more cost-effective than malaria control.[221] Given the current funding climate, efforts are probably better directed at control than elimination or eradication for the near-term.

Still, many experts are beginning to advocate that malaria can be eliminated from Africa, a goal that was unthinkable even a few years ago — and that LLINs are perhaps the major reason for this.[222] Many signs indicate renewed progress in the global fight against malaria. ITNs/LLINs are clearly a major factor, and with continued advocacy, funding, and control efforts, much progress can be made. While new interventions (such as a malaria vaccine) may be needed to bring eradication within reach, vector control measures including ITNs/LLINs remain crucial to malaria control efforts in the meantime.[7,223] The full potential of these remarkably cost-effective control measures remains to be seen, and ITNs/LLINs may soon help with achievement of the ambitious goals of decreasing malaria mortality

---

[221] Zanzibar Malaria Control Program, Malaria elimination in Zanzibar: a feasibility assessment, 2009, 7–10: Zanzibar, Tanzania.

[222] C.C. Campbell and R.W. Steketee, Malaria in Africa can be eliminated, *American Journal of Tropical Medicine and Hygiene*, 2011, **85**(4), 584–5.

[223] K. Mendis *et al.*, From malaria control to eradication: the WHO perspective, *Tropical Medicine and International Health*, 2009, **14**(7), 802–9.

by half and the broader Millennium Development Goal of reducing U5 mortality by two-thirds. While much progress remains before the ambitious coverage targets set during this past decade are reached, a renewed hope exists that they may be obtainable, and result in continued and substantial progress in the global fight against malaria.

8 The Scientific and Medical Challenge of Malaria

Tiffany Sun and Richard Bucala

Introduction

Adequate control, if not the eradication of malaria, is a pressing global health goal. Perhaps the greatest scientific and medical challenge of malaria is the development of an anti-malaria vaccine that can help achieve worldwide malaria control.

Not only have we been unable to develop an efficacious vaccine, but the characteristics of a protective anti-malaria immune response remain unknown. Since malaria parasites invade red blood cells, virtually all organs and cells of the host are exposed to malaria antigens, and the scientific community of malaria researchers is actively investigating all arms of the immune response. Many groups have provided valuable information on how individual components of the immune system respond to malaria infection, but the 'optimal' response to malaria infection — the response needed for parasite clearance, host survival, and long term immunity — remains unclear. This chapter focuses on the host immune response during malaria infection. We describe the current state of malaria research by consolidating current knowledge and highlighting key obstacles in vaccine development.

Parasite Life Cycle

Malaria is a vector-borne disease that is transmitted between humans by mosquitoes. Currently, five known species of *Plasmodium* parasites cause malaria in humans: *P. ovale*, *P. malariae*, *P. vivax*, *P. falciparum*, and *P. knowlesi*. The devastating global health impact of malaria was long thought to be caused mostly by *P. falciparum*, with lesser contributions by *P. vivax*; however, recent reports suggest that *P. knowlesi*, previously believed to infect non-human primate hosts, has adapted to the human host and causes *P. falciparum*-like symptoms.[1] The World Health Organization currently estimates that malaria affects nearly 250 million people yearly, killing close to 1 million people, mostly children.[2]

The *Plasmodium* parasite begins its life cycle as a sporozoite form that resides in the mosquito midgut. Once sporozoites mature, they migrate to the salivary glands of the mosquito and are then injected into the host when the mosquito inserts its proboscis into the skin to take a bloodmeal. In one bite, 10–100 sporozoites are inoculated into the host.[3] The final destination for the sporozoites is the host liver, but the route and time taken to get to the liver remains a focus of investigation and debate. Some studies report that the sporozoites travel directly to the liver through the circulation, arriving there within minutes, while others indicate that sporozoites meander in the dermis close to the site of injection for 1–6 hours after the bite before migrating to the liver. Further reports also suggest that some sporozoites take a detour, via the lymphatics, to the lymph node draining the site of infection.[4] It is uncertain whether the lymph node sporozoites eventually reach in the liver.

Debating the time required for sporozoites to reach the liver may seem trivial but knowing how long the human host is exposed to sporozoite proteins is in fact crucial for vaccine development. Since most anti-malaria vaccine candidates developed so far are based on eliciting an anti-sporozoite response, the sporozoite antigens must remain exposed to immune cells for an adequate length of time in order for the vaccine to be effective. If sporozoites persist in the dermis for several hours, then sentinel immune cells can sample sporozoite proteins and activate adaptive immune cells to mount a protective response. In this case, sporozoite proteins are plausible candidates for inducing protective immunity because memory responses against these protein antigens will have sufficient time to kill the sporozoites before the parasites migrate into the liver during a subsequent infection. Likewise, if sporozoites travel to lymph nodes, they may be able to activate resident memory cells before the parasites reach the blood stage. In contrast, if all sporozoites enter hepatocytes within minutes, it is unlikely that sporozoites proteins circulate long enough to elicit a robust immune response. Even if memory responses against the sporozoites are established, several minutes is probably an inadequate

[1]J. Cox-Singh *et al.*, *Plasmodium knowlesi* malaria in humans is widely distributed and potentially life threatening, *Clinical Infectious Diseases*, 2008, **46**(2), 165–71.

[2]WHO, World Health Organization Malaria, 2008 [cited; Available from: http://www.who.int/topics/malaria/en/.

[3]M.M. Stevenson and E.M. Riley, Innate immunity to malaria, *Nature Reviews Immunology*, 2004, **4**(3), 169–80.

[4]R. Amino *et al.*, Quantitative imaging of *Plasmodium* transmission from mosquito to mammal, *Nature Medicine*, 2006, **12**(2), 220–4.

amount of time for the activation of memory cells to protect against another infection.

Once sporozoites reach the liver, they must be activated before infecting a hepatocyte. The activation process involves migrating through several hepatocytes and possibly epithelial cells before infecting a single hepatocyte. For the parasite, migrating through hepatocytes without infection may protect the sporozoites from detection by resident macrophages,[5] but plasma membrane damage caused by the migrations also serves as one of the first signs of invasion.[6] In the infected hepatocyte, sporozoites develop and multiply into the exoerythrocytic form of the parasite. After 1–2 weeks of residing inside hepatocytes, the exoerythrocytic forms become merozoites and rupture the hepatocytes. Upon rupture, thousands of parasites in the merozoites form are released into the host circulation.

Merozoites and their progeny exclusively infect mature and immature red blood cells. The red blood cell invasion process is a tightly coordinated sequence of events that involve both host and parasite surface proteins. Proteolytic processing of several proteins, such as MSP-1, which is at the apical end of the parasite must occur immediately prior to entry. The cleaved subunits of MSP-1 do not enter the red blood cell and may become immunogenic in the circulation.[7,8] The parasite takes part of the red blood cell membrane during entry to form a parasitophorus vacuole[9] and the merozoite matures into the ring and trophozoite stages from within the vacuole contained inside the infected red blood cell. During the ring and trophozoite stages, the parasite completely remodels the architecture of the red blood cell to suit its pathogenic and nutritional needs. Numerous parasite products are synthesized and secreted into the cytosol and surface of the red blood cell, while many red blood cell proteins, such as hemoglobin, are degraded.[10] Some parasite products aid in sequestration of the infected red blood cells from the host immune system and others modulate the host response, but how these products are

---

[5]R. Amino *et al.*, Host cell traversal is important for progression of the malaria parasite through the dermis to the liver, *Cell Host and Microbe*, 2008, **3**(2), 88–96.

[6]M.M. Mota *et al.*, Migration of *Plasmodium sporozoites* through cells before infection, *Science*, 2001, **291**(5501), 141–4.

[7]M.J. Blackman *et al.*, Proteolytic processing of the *Plasmodium falciparum* merozoite surface protein-1 produces a membrane-bound fragment containing two epidermal growth factor-like domains, *Molecular and Biochemical Parasitology*, 1991, **49**(1), 29–33.

[8]R.A. O'Donnell *et al.*, Intramembrane proteolysis mediates shedding of a key adhesin during erythrocyte invasion by the malaria parasite, *Journal of Cell Biology*, 2006, **174**(7), 1023–33.

[9]K. Lingelbachand K.A. Joiner, The parasitophorous vacuole membrane surrounding *Plasmodium* and *Toxoplasma*: an unusual compartment in infected cells, *Journal of Cell Science*, 1998, **111**(11), 1467–75.

[10]K. Haldar *et al.*, Protein and lipid trafficking induced in erythrocytes infected by malaria parasites, *Cell Microbiology*, 2002, **4**(7), 383–95.

trafficked and secreted remains unclear. One important parasite product that is formed in the infected red blood cell is hemozoin, which appears to alter the host immune response to infection. After the trophozoite matures, it undergoes schizogony, during which 16–32 daughter merozoites are formed. Approximately 48 hours after the initial red blood cell infection, the daughter merozoites burst the infected red blood cell and become free merozoites.[11]

When the merozoites rupture the infected red blood cell, the merozoites and all the parasite proteins once contained within the infected red blood cell are exposed to the full gamut of the host immune system. Since the blood stage parasites are well synchronized in human malaria, the host is suddenly exposed to an enormous malaria antigen load. The host responds by inducing a highly inflammatory state marked by fevers and chills, and in the case of *falciparum* malaria, these symptoms recur every two days, after each round of schizogony. The pathologies associated with malaria, including cerebral malaria, severe anemia, lactic acidosis, renal failure, and sepsis, thus occurs during the blood stage of infection.[11]

Detection of Infection

Once malaria sporozoites mature and divide into merozoites within the infected hepatocyte, the parasites burst from the infected cell and enter into the host circulation by infecting red blood cells. After entry into a red blood cell, the malaria parasite promptly begins to hijack nutrients and machinery from the host cell to create a suitable environment for parasite development. The parasite uses the host red blood cell both as a source of essential nutrients and as a means of concealment from the immune system.[12] One major mechanism of subverting the immune system is that malaria exclusively invades red blood cells, the only cells that do not express Major Histocompatibility Complex Class I (MHC class I) proteins. Normally, humans rely heavily on presentation of foreign antigens on MHC class I to detect infection, but this does not occur in the case of malaria-infected red cells.

Upon infection, the parasite remodels the infected red blood cell by secreting approximately 8% of its entire proteome into the cytosol and trafficking many of these parasite proteins onto the surface of the red blood cell.[13] One of the proteins secreted onto the surface of the infected red blood cell is the variable *P. falciparum* Erythrocyte Membrane Protein-1 (PfEMP-1, homologues are found in other malarial species), which makes the infected red blood cell 'sticky'. PfEMP can bind to

---

[11]L. Schofield and G.E. Grau, Immunological processes in malaria pathogenesis, *Nature Reviews Immunology*, 2005, **5**(9), 722–35.

[12]M. Marti *et al.*, Targeting malaria virulence and remodeling proteins to the host erythrocyte, *Science*, 2004, **306**(5703), 1930–3.

[13]S. Roetynck*et al.*, Natural killer cells and malaria, *Immunological Reviews*, 2006, **214**, 251–63.

uninfected red blood cell surfaces, resulting in a cluster of normal red blood cells concealing an infected red blood cell in the middle. PfEMP also can bind to endothelial cells via Intracellular Adhesion Molecule-1 (ICAM-1), which allows the infected red blood cell to be sequestered in the microvasculature deep inside tissues.[14] Remodeling the infected red blood cell does not occur without consequences to the parasite. Although upregulation of PfEMP-1 allows the infected red blood cell to adhere to the endothelium via binding to ICAM-1, PfEMP-1 can also bind CD36, a scavenger receptor on macrophages and dendritic cells. Bound CD36 on macrophages triggers receptor-mediated endocytosis, and the infected red blood cell is internalized into the macrophage.[14] Endocytosis results in parasite killing,[15] and upregulation of innate immune sensors such as toll-like receptors (TLRs). By itself, CD36-mediated endocytosis is not pro-inflammatory, but can augment TLR expression and synergistically increase inflammatory cytokine production.[16]

The mammalian innate immune response recognizes molecular patterns of pathogens that are largely conserved. These molecular patterns occur commonly among different pathogens but their structural motifs differ significantly from those that occur in host molecules. Several classes of innate immune pattern recognition proteins are found in humans; the ones relevant to malaria recognition are the toll-like receptors (TLRs) and the nod-like receptors (NLRs).[17] Many cells express TLRs and NLRs, but both are most highly expressed by antigen presenting cells like macrophages and dendritic cells. TLRs are expressed on the cell surface and in endosomes to detect extracellular and phagocytosed pathogens,[18] and NLRs are found in the cytosol to detect intracellular infections.[19] Signaling through either TLRs and NLRs result in inflammation; TLR signaling induces the activation of transcription factors that upregulate expression of inflammatory cytokines[18] while NLR signaling results in the activation and secretion of IL-1β and IL-18.[19]

TLR signaling during malaria infection has not been completely elucidated. Experimental malaria infections of mice lacking MyD88, an adaptor molecule

[14]B.C. Urban and D.J. Roberts, Malaria, monocytes, macrophages and myeloid dendritic cells: sticking of infected erythrocytes switches off host cells, *Current Opinion in Immunology*, 2002, **14**(4), 458–65.

[15]B.J. Angus *et al.*, *In vivo* removal of malaria parasites from red blood cells without their destruction in acute *falciparum* malaria, *Blood*, 1997, **90**(5), 2037–40.

[16]L.K. Erdman *et al.*, CD36 and TLR interactions in inflammation and phagocytosis: implications for malaria, *Journal of Immunology*, 2009, **183**(10), 6452–9.

[17]E. Meylan, J. Tschopp and M. Karin, Intracellular pattern recognition receptors in the host response, *Nature*, 2006, **442**(7098), 39–44.

[18]C.A. Janeway Jr. and R. Medzhitov, Innate immune recognition. *Annual Review of Immunology*, 2002, **20**, 197–216.

[19]F. Martinon and J. Tschopp, NLRs join TLRs as innate sensors of pathogens, *Trends in Immunology*, 2005, **26**(8), 447–54.

through which the TLR signal is transmitted, demonstrated that inflammatory cytokine production is decreased in the absence of MyD88.[20,21] These observations suggest that one or more TLRs contribute to the detection of malaria infection. Using macrophages isolated from various TLR knockout mice, Krishnegowda *et al.* showed that the malaria surface product glycosylphosphatidylinositol (GPI) is recognized predominately by TLR2 and by TLR4 to a lesser extent. GPI is commonly found on eukaryotic cells, including host cells, as a means of anchoring proteins to the plasma membrane, but the structure of mammalian GPI differs significantly from malarial GPI, allowing for detection by TLR2.[22] Signaling of GPI through TLR2 causes increased secretion of TNF-α as well as phosphorylation of MAP kinase components, resulting in activation of NF-κB[23] and downstream inflammation. Additionally, macrophage phospholipases can cleave the phosphatidylinositol portion of malarial GPI, rendering it inactive.

Signaling through TLR2/4 does not account for the entire difference in cytokine production between wildtype and *MyD88-/-*infections, suggesting the involvement of other TLRs. Infection of *Tlr9-/-*mice also showed decreased production of inflammatory cytokines, however the malaria products detected by TLR9 remain controversial.[24,25] TLR9 is an intracellular toll-like receptor that is expressed in endosomes and was first described to detect unmethylated CpG DNA, which is a feature of prokaryotic organisms.[26] Several groups showed that the malarial byproduct hemozoin activates TLR9 signaling[25] while others have argued that pure hemozoin is immunologically inert.[27] Hemozoin is a byproduct of malarial heme

---

[20]J.W. Griffith *et al.*, Toll-like receptor modulation of murine cerebral malaria is dependent on the genetic background of the host, *Journal of Infectious Diseases*, 2007, **196**(10), 1553–64.

[21]K. Adachi *et al.*, *Plasmodium berghei* infection in mice induces liver injury by an IL-12- and toll-like receptor/myeloid differentiation factor 88-dependent mechanism, *Journal of Immunology*, 2001, 167(10), 5928–34.

[22]C. Coban *et al.*, Manipulation of host innate immune responses by the malaria parasite, *Trends in Microbiology*, 2007, **15**(6), 271–8.

[23]G. Krishnegowda *et al.*, Induction of proinflammatory responses in macrophages by the glycosylphosphatidylinositols of *Plasmodium falciparum*: cell signaling receptors, glycosylphosphatidylinositol (GPI) structural requirement, and regulation of GPI activity, *Journal of Biology and Chemistry*, 2005, **280**(9), 8606–16.

[24]S. Pichyangkul *et al.*, Malaria blood stage parasites activate human plasmacytoid dendritic cells and murine dendritic cells through a Toll-like receptor 9-dependent pathway, *Journal of Immunology*, 2004, **172**(8), 4926–33.

[25]C. Coban *et al.*, Toll-like receptor 9 mediates innate immune activation by the malaria pigment hemozoin, *Journal of Experimental Medicine*, 2005, **201**(1), 19–25.

[26]H. Hemmi *et al.*, A Toll-like receptor recognizes bacterial DNA, *Nature*, 2000, **408**(6813), 740–5.

[27]P. Parroche *et al.*, Malaria hemozoin is immunologically inert but radically enhances innate responses by presenting malaria DNA to Toll-like receptor 9. *Proceedings of the National Academy of Sciences of the United States of America*, 2007, **104**(6), 1919–24.

detoxification that accumulates in the infected red blood cell. Hemozoin is released into circulation upon infected red blood cell rupture and it is readily taken up by macrophages and dendritic cells, but the inflammatory properties of hemozoin remain unclear. Hemozoin may act as a carrier for malaria DNA, which can stimulate TLR9 within the endosome.[27] It also has been suggested that TLR9 is activated by malaria DNA together with an unknown malaria protein.[22] The downstream effects of hemozoin signaling also remain controversial. Research groups have alternately shown hemozoin to be inflammatory,[25] inert,[27] or suppressive for APC function.[28,29]

Recent research on the innate immune response to malaria has focused on another class of pattern recognition receptors, the Nod-like receptors (NLRs). Studies of malaria infection in mice with various components of NLR signaling proteins genetically knocked out suggest that NLRs are partially responsible for detection of blood stage infection. It appears that the NLR sensor, NALP3, detects either a parasite product, likely hemozoin, or injury caused by malaria infection, likely uric acid release.[30]

Yet another malaria-derived product that is recognized by the immune system is the microparticle (MP). MPs are vesicular blebbings derived from the plasma membrane when cells are undergoing activation or apoptosis. Couper *et al.* demonstrated that MPs obtained from malaria-infected cells can activate macrophages much more efficiently than MPs from uninfected cells. The host sensor for MP detection has not been identified, but it appears to occur in a TLR-independent manner. MPs from infected red blood cells induce upregulation of surface activation markers in macrophages and increase secretion of TNF-α.[31]

Macrophages

Macrophages are abundant antigen presenting cells that play multiple roles during the blood stage of malaria infection. They sense parasites in the host bloodstream and respond by phagocytosing the invaders and by activating other components of the host immune system.

---

[28] B.C. Urban and S. Todryk, Malaria pigment paralyzes dendritic cells, *Journal of Biology*, 2006, **5**(2), 4.

[29] E. Schwarzer *et al.*, Phagocytosis of the malarial pigment, hemozoin, impairs expression of major histocompatibility complex class II antigen, CD54, and CD11c in human monocytes, *Infection and Immunity*, 1998, **66**(4), 1601–6.

[30] J.W. Griffith *et al.*, Pure Hemozoin is inflammatory *in vivo* and activates the NALP3 inflammasome via release of uric acid, *Journal of Immunology*, 2009, **183**(8), 5208–20.

[31] K.N. Couper *et al.*, Parasite-derived plasma microparticles contribute significantly to malaria infection-induced inflammation through potent macrophage stimulation, *Public Library of Science Pathogens*, **6**(1), e1000744.

Macrophages are activated upon detection or phagocytosis of parasites by the mechanisms discussed above, and they can also undergo antigen-independent activation by cytokines such as interferon gamma (IFN-γ). Macrophages are highly sensitive to IFN-γ secreted by activated NK cells and T cells during infection, and they respond to IFN-γ by upregulating expression of inducible nitric oxide synthase (iNOS) and increasing NO production.[3]

Once macrophages detect malaria infection and become activated, they can induce systemic inflammation and activate other innate immune cells, kill parasites, and present malaria antigens to cells of the adaptive immune response. Macrophages that have engulfed infected red blood cells can efficiently kill parasites by inducing the nitric oxide synthase gene, thereby increasing nitric oxide production. Nitric oxide kills the parasite by depriving it of iron and it can also directly inhibit malaria enzymes.[32] It is likely that in the majority of cases, the red blood cell is destroyed when parasites are killed, but Angus *et al.* showed that macrophages may also 'pit' the parasite from the red blood cell, thus extending the lifespan of the previously infected red blood cell.[15]

Another mechanism of parasite recognition and killing is through the macrophage's Fc receptors. Fc receptors on the macrophage surface bind the constant region of antibodies, and signaling through the bound antibody elicits a semi-specific pathogen response. Upon binding of malarial antigens to the macrophage-bound antibody, the macrophage is activated to secrete malarial inhibitors. Interestingly the malaria inhibitors, which have not been molecularly identified, appear to exclusively block nuclear division of the parasites.[33] This is a significant finding because it suggests that the human immune system has evolved to recognize efficient ways to rid the body of parasites. Activated macrophages also upregulate their TLRs for increased parasite detection and surveillance.

Macrophages activated by the engulfment of parasites kill the parasites and cleave parasite proteins into short peptides. These peptides are then loaded onto either Major Histocompatibility Complex (MHC) Class I or II molecules and transported to the cell surface. The expression of co-stimulatory molecules such as CD40, CD80 and CD86, are increased to aid presentation of malaria antigen to T cells. Furthermore, activated macrophages rapidly secrete the cytokines TNF-α and IL-12,[34] which potently induce systemic inflammation and activate other immune cells to respond to the infection.

---

[32] S.L. James, Role of nitric oxide in parasitic infections. *Microbiological Reviews*, 1995, **59**(4), 533–47.

[33] H. Bouharoun-Tayoun *et al.*, Mechanisms underlying the monocyte-mediated antibody-dependent killing of *Plasmodium falciparum* asexual blood stages, *Journal of Experimental Medicine*, 1995, **182**(2), 409–18.

[34] A. Horowitz *et al.*, Cross-talk between T cells and NK cells generates rapid effector responses to *Plasmodium falciparum*-infected erythrocytes, *Journal of Immunology,* 2010, **184**(11), 6043–52.

Dendritic Cells

Dendritic cells are specialized antigen presenting cells that patrol the peripheral environment by frequently sampling antigens. These cells are highly phagocytic and endocytosed antigens are processed into short peptides that are subsequently presented on the cell surface in a complex with an MHC class II molecule. Once dendritic cells detect foreign antigen, they upregulate expression of costimulatory molecules and travel to the spleen or lymph nodes to present the foreign antigen and activate antigen-specific T cells. T cells can only be activated by dendritic cells that express both the antigen-MHC class I complex and co-stimulatory molecules. In this way, dendritic cells are the most direct link between the innate and adaptive immune systems. Dendritic cells also increase their secretion of inflammatory cytokines, especially IL-12, to further activate NK cells and macrophages.[3]

The manner by which dendritic cells detect antigen is very similar to that of macrophages. Dendritic cells express the same TLRs, CD36 and other potential malaria antigen receptors as macrophages but at a higher expression level, making dendritic cells more efficient at detecting infection.[3] However, the increased efficiency with which dendritic cells are able to phagocytose and sample antigen also renders them more vulnerable to parasite-induced immunosuppression. The degree to which malaria parasites can dampen the host immune response by hindering the antigen presentation process is highly controversial. Early malaria researchers compared the ability of adherent splenocytes (presumably macrophages and dendritic cells) from uninfected and from malaria-infected mice to take up equine red blood cells and observed that antigen presentation was impaired during malaria infection.[35] More recently, Urban *et al.* reported that after stimulating dendritic cells with high ratios of *P. falciparum*-infected red blood cells, dendritic cells enter a 'paralyzed' state, as measured by the failure to upregulate surface co-stimulatory molecules and the inability to stimulate T cells.[36] Hemozoin was later implicated as the malarial metabolite that impairs dendritic cells.[37] A contrasting view of dendritic cell suppression by infected red blood cells was demonstrated in a *P. chabaudi* mouse infection model. In this study, dendritic cells were found to be fully functional for migrating to and activating T cells, even during peak parasite loads. One defect of dendritic cells observed in the *P. chabaudi*

[35]H.S. Warren and W.P. Weidanz, Malarial immunodepression *in vitro*: adherent spleen cells are functionally defective as accessory cells in the response to horse erythrocytes. *European Journal of Immunology*, 1976, **6**(11), 816–9.

[36]B.C. Urban *et al.*, *Plasmodium falciparum*-infected erythrocytes modulate the maturation of dendritic cells, *Nature*, 1999, **400**(6739), 73–7.

[37]O.A. Skorokhod *et al.*, Hemozoin (malarial pigment) inhibits differentiation and maturation of human monocyte-derived dendritic cells: a peroxisome proliferator-activated receptor-gamma-mediated effect, *Journal of Immunology*, 2004, **173**(6), 4066–74.

experiment was that T cells did not cluster well around dendritic cells, which could explain the reduced proliferation of T cells.[38]

Dendritic cell function during malaria infection is sensitive to a variety of parameters. The type of dendritic cell that is activated, the antigen dose, and the time course of dendritic cell activation all appear to affect the dendritic cell response. Many different subsets of dendritic cells exist, and each subset acts differently in response to an antigen. Throughout infection, signaling through conventional dendritic cells tends to mediate protection and parasite killing whereas plasmacytoid dendritic cells favor a Th2 response that supports viable parasites.[39] Further work is needed to identify and characterize dendritic cell subsets. Wykes *et al.* also found that the strain of parasite can impact dendritic cell function. Infections with the lethal and non-lethal strains of *P. yoelii* showed that dendritic cells were fully functional, but dendritic cells isolated from mice infected with the lethal strain showed deficiencies in antigen presentation, costimulatory molecule expression, and secretion of TNFα and IL-12.[40] Antigen dose, measured by parasite burden, is another factor in enhancement or impairment of dendritic cell function.[41] Dendritic cell function during malaria infection is also temporally regulated. During early malaria infection, only CD8- subsets of dendritic cells are capable of activating T cells, but as infection progresses, dendritic cells become less able to produce IL-12 and TNF-α, and some populations of dendritic cells begin to apoptose.[42] Sustained levels of inflammatory cytokines like TNF-α also contributes to the inhibition of dendritic cell function.[43]

Natural Killer (NK) Cells

Natural killer cells play an important role in the complex network of immune effector cells during bloodstage malaria infection. The necessity for adequate levels of IFN-γ in malaria infection has long been appreciated, and Stevenson *et al.*

[38]O.R. Millington *et al.*, Malaria impairs T cell clustering and immune priming despite normal signal 1 from dendritic cells, *Public Library of Science Pathogens*, 2007, **3**(10), 1380–7.

[39]K.A. Wongand A. Rodriguez, *Plasmodium* infection and endotoxic shock induce the expansion of regulatory dendritic cells, *Journal of Immunology*, 2008, **180**(2), 716–26.

[40]M.N. Wykes *et al.*, Plasmodium strain determines dendritic cell function essential for survival from malaria, *Public Library of Science Pathogens*, 2007, **3**(7), e96.

[41]M.N. Wykes and M.F. Good, What really happens to dendritic cells during malaria?, *Nature Reviews Microbiology*, 2008, **6**(11), 864–70.

[42]A.M. Sponaas *et al.*, Malaria infection changes the ability of splenic dendritic cell populations to stimulate antigen-specific T cells, *Journal of Experimental Medicine*, 2006, **203**(6), 1427–33.

[43]J.A. Perry *et al.*, Cutting edge: the acquisition of TLR tolerance during malaria infection impacts T cell activation, *Journal of Immunology*, 2005, **174**(10), 5921–5.

established that the main producers of IFN-γ during early bloodstage infection were not Th1 T cells, but rather NK cells.[44]

Unlike macrophages and dendritic cells, NK cells are not professional antigen presenting cells and thus are not readily activated by endocytosis of parasite products. NK cells alone can detect infected red blood cells and become activated to secrete cytokines, however these cells require macrophage help via IL-18 and possibly IL-12 to become fully activated.[45] Recently, Horowitz *et al.* showed that NK cells also require IL-2 from antigen-exposed T cells to be able to secrete IFN-γ.[34] NK cells have been observed to form rosettes with infected red blood cells but not uninfected red blood cells, suggesting that NK cells express a malaria-specific receptor;[46,47] however, the receptor has yet to be identified.

As a consequence of both increased proliferation and mobilization from organs such as the spleen, the number of NK cells increase transiently in the peripheral blood in response to the release of merozoites from the liver. Activated NK cells can simultaneously induce IFN-γ production and mediate parasiticidal activity in as little as two hours under *in vitro* conditions.[34] NK cells are the main producers of IFN-γ early during infection, before antigen presentation to Th1 T cells can occur, and the secreted IFN-γ activates macrophages to produce NO in a positive feedback loop. In addition to IFN-γ secretion, NK cells also release the inflammatory cytokines and chemokines TNF-α, IL-13, GM-CSF, MIP-1α, MIP-1β, CCL5 and RANTES. An early robust IFN-γ response has been shown to reduce fever and clinical malaria symptoms, but high, sustained levels of IFN-γ which ultimately leads to severe immunopathology.[47,48]

Additionally, NK cells can be directly cytotoxic to malaria parasites by upregulating the Klr (lectin-like killer cell receptor) genes and inducing apoptosis.[49] The role of NK cells in controlling parasite replication was confirmed in models of

[44] K. Mohan, P. Moulin and M.M. Stevenson, Natural killer cell cytokine production, not cytotoxicity, contributes to resistance against blood-stage *Plasmodium chabaudi* AS infection, *Journal of Immunology*, 1997, **159**(10), 4990–8.

[45] K. Artavanis-Tsakonas *et al.*, Activation of a subset of human NK cells upon contact with *Plasmodium falciparum*-infected erythrocytes, *Journal of Immunology*, 2003, **171**(10), 5396–405.

[46] K. Artavanis-Tsakonas and E.M. Riley, Innate immune response to malaria: rapid induction of IFN-gamma from human NK cells by live *Plasmodium falciparum*-infected erythrocytes, *Journal of Immunology*, 2002, **169**(6), 2956–63.

[47] M. Baratin *et al.*, Natural killer cell and macrophage cooperation in MyD88-dependent innate responses to *Plasmodium falciparum*. *Proceedings of the National Academy of Sciences of the United States of America*, 2005, **102**(41), 14747–52.

[48] H.C. van der Heyde *et al.*, The time course of selected malarial infections in cytokine-deficient mice, *Experimental Parasitology*, 1997, **85**(2), 206–13.

[49] C.C. Kim *et al.*, Experimental malaria infection triggers early expansion of natural killer cells, *Infection and Immunity*, 2008, **76**(12), 5873–82.

experimental malaria using *Plasmodium chabaudi* AS to infect wildtype and NK cell-depleted mice. *P. chabaudi* infection of wildtype mice results in one peak of parasitemia that is subsequently controlled during the acute phase and eliminated during the chronic phase. In contrast, *P. chabaudi* infection of NK cell-depleted mice results in a higher peak of parasitemia during the acute phase, followed by a second wave of parasitemia during the chronic phase.[44]

NK cell dependence on the cytokines IL-18 and IL-12 for full activation inextricably links this innate immune cell to other components of the innate immune response, namely macrophages and dendritic cells. In turn, macrophages are equally reliant on IFN-γ produced by the NK cells for activation and induction of NO-mediated parasite killing. Moreover, chemokines secreted by NK cells guide the innate and adaptive immune cells to sites of infection.[50]

γδ T Cells

T cells that express the γδ TCR chains make up a small portion of the T cell population and have not been extensively characterized. These T cells appear to bridge the innate and the adaptive immune cell populations. On one hand, γδ T cells have potent antigen presenting capabilities and detect pathogens via pattern recognition receptors; on the other hand, γδ T cell effector responses can skew towards a Th1 or Th2 response in a similar manner as CD4 T cells.[51] During malaria infection, γδ T cells have been implicated in playing anywhere from a major role to a non-relevant role in the immune response.

Studies of the role of γδ T cells during malaria infection suggest that γδ T cells contribute to inflammation and are tightly regulated temporally. D'Ombrain *et al.* found that γδ T cells produce the majority of the circulating IFN-γ by characterizing subsets of PBMCs that release IFN-γ after stimulation with *P. falciparum*-infected red blood cells.[52] While some investigators suggest that γδ T cells do indeed produce IFN-γ during malaria infection,[52] others contend that γδ T cells produce only minor amounts of IFN-γ and instead contribute significantly to inflammation by producing a second burst of TNF-α (after macrophages make the initial burst).[34] These contrasting findings may not be mutually exclusive when one

[50]R. Ing. and M.M. Stevenson, Dendritic cell and NK cell reciprocal cross talk promotes gamma interferon-dependent immunity to blood-stage *Plasmodium chabaudi* AS infection in mice, *Infection and Immunity*, 2009, **77**(2), 770–82.

[51]M. Bonneville, R.L. O'Brien, and W.K. Born, Gammadelta T cell effector functions: a blend of innate programming and acquired plasticity, *Nature Reviews Immunology,* 2010 **10**(7), 467–78.

[52]M.C. D'Ombrain *et al.*, Gammadelta-T cells expressing NK receptors predominate over NK cells and conventional T cells in the innate IFN-gamma response to *Plasmodium falciparum* malaria, *European Journal of Immunology*, 2007, **37**(7), 1864–73.

notes that the actions of γδ T cells appear to occur within a narrow time frame, and experimental results may vary depending on the time course of measurements taken during *in vitro* stimulations and on the progression of disease in the different malaria mouse models.

Adaptive Immunity

The age-old conundrum of malaria is the inability of the host to maintain immunity. Unlike most other infections in which a single exposure affords long-lived protection, humans remain continually susceptible to malaria re-infection. Two possible explanations for why humans are perpetually susceptible are that protective responses are not formed or that immunity wanes quickly without frequent re-stimulation by malaria antigens. It also remains unknown whether the humoral or the cellular response or (more likely) both are responsible for the inadequate immunity.

Although naturally-acquired sterile immunity to malaria has never been documented, the adaptive immune response is not an idle bystander during malaria infection. All components of the adaptive immune system are activated by the malaria parasites at various stages of infection and most likely some immunologic memory of a previous infection is retained.

The adaptive immune response refers to antigen-specific responses that are induced by CD4 T cells, CD8 T cells or B cells. The cells of the adaptive immune system express receptors that recognize short peptides of specific antigens. Two unique features of T cell and B cell receptors are that they can undergo somatic hypermutation to increase affinity for an antigen, and cells with high affinity receptors can develop into memory cells that persist for years, perhaps even for life. Recognition of an antigen by a specific T or B cell receptor results in the induction of a rapid and potent cascade of anti-pathogen responses. To protect against autoimmunity, activation of adaptive immune cells is highly regulated. T and B cells can only recognize antigen presented as part of a specific MHC protein complex by antigen presenting cells. T and B cells must also receive a second stimulatory signal from co-stimulatory molecules to be fully activated.[53]

CD4 T Cells

CD4 T cells comprise a major arm of the adaptive immune system. During malaria infection, malaria specific CD4 T cells are generally primed in the spleen and once

---

[53]J. Langhorne *et al.*, Dendritic cells, pro-inflammatory responses, and antigen presentation in a rodent malaria infection, *Immunological Reviews*, 2004, **201**, 35–47.

activated, CD4 T cell can coordinate a systemic inflammatory (Th1) or non-inflammatory (Th2) response. The adaptive immune system relies on CD4 T cells for parasite detection. CD8 T cells are unable to detect blood stage malaria parasites because CD8 T cells only recognize antigens presented by MHC class I, which are not expressed on human red blood cells.[54] CD4 T cells recognize antigen presented on MHC class II proteins, which are expressed primarily by antigen presenting cells (APCs). When APCs encounter foreign particles, they process the antigen, load the processed antigens on MHC class II proteins, and express this combination on the cell surface. Simultaneously with antigen processing and presentation, APCs travel to T cell rich areas such as the spleen and lymph nodes to present these foreign particles to pathogen-specific T cells, thereby activating the adaptive immune response.[53] Once malaria-specific T cells encounter cognate antigen, the T cells proliferate and secrete a panel of cytokines. Among the cytokines secreted, IL-2 acts in a paracrine manner to further increase proliferation, and IFN-γ and IL-4 differentiates between Th1 and Th2 CD4 T cells, respectively.[11] Upon pathogen clearance, a dramatic contraction phase follows CD4 T cell expansion. At the conclusion of this phase, a few cells with high affinity receptors for the pathogen remain as memory cells with low steady state replication.[55]

The importance of CD4 T cells in the development of malarial immunity was first demonstrated in the *P. chabaudi* mouse model of malaria infection. Tsuji *et al.* derived malaria specific CD4 T cell clones by immunizing mice with irradiated sporozoites. The CD4 T cells were then adoptively transferred and the recipient mouse was infected. Although the transferred CD4 T cells did not recognize the immunodominant sporozoite protein, they strongly recognized blood stage antigens. Surprisingly, the transferred cells conferred protection against sprozoite challenge, but not against blood stage infection.[56] Further studies revealed that both Th1 and Th2 T cell clones can be anti-parasitic. Th1 T cells responsive to malaria antigen induced a IFN-γ mediated-, NO-dependent protection, while Th2 CD4 T cells secrete IL-4, which promotes B cell production of high affinity anti-malaria antibodies.[57] It should be noted that recent studies suggest that these

---

[54]M.F. Good *et al.*, The immunological challenge to developing a vaccine to the blood stages of malaria parasites, *Immunological Reviews*, 2004, **201**, 254–67.

[55]S.M. Kaech, E.J. Wherry and R. Ahmed, Effect or and memory T-cell differentiation: implications for vaccine development, *Nature Reviews Immunology*, 2002, **2**(4), 251–62.

[56]M. Tsuji *et al.*, CD4+ cytolytic T cell clone confers protection against murine malaria, *Journal of Experimental Medicine*, 1990, **172**(5), 1353–7.

[57]A.W. Taylor-Robinson *et al.*, The role of TH1 and TH2 cells in a rodent malaria infection, *Science*, 1993, **260**(5116), 1931–4.

IL-4-secreting CD4 T cells may in fact be classified as T follicular helper cells (Tfh) rather than Th2 cells.[58]

Once activated, malaria-specific CD4 T cells are the main cellular source of sustained IFN-γ production, which induces NO-mediated parasite killing.[59] Even though the IFN-γ-secreting Th1 T cells are believed to be vital for parasite clearance, they must be tightly coordinated to prevent excessive inflammation and death. Cerebral malaria is likely caused by activated macrophages in the brain that induce a highly inflammatory state that leads to paralysis, coma and death.[60] Repeated exposure to low numbers of parasites appears to be optimal for the activation and expansion of CD4 T cells. Volunteers who were infected periodically with "ultra-low" dose of parasites (about 30 infected red blood cells) generated T cells that could efficiently proliferate, secrete IFN-γ, and induce nitric oxide production *in vitro* in response to malaria antigen. CD4 T cells generated from the low infection doses also seem to afford lasting protection, suggesting that cellular immunological memory against malaria infection can indeed be attained.[61] Further in depth studies on the immune response to very low doses of parasites could offer valuable insight into the nature of protective immunity to malaria.

Unlike most infections in which pathogen-specific T cells undergo expansion followed by contraction to establish a small pool of memory T cells with high affinity for the pathogen, malaria infection appears to induce complete contraction of all antigen-specific T cells. Inflammation during the acute phase of the blood-stage infection causes increased apoptosis and depletes malaria-specific CD4 T cells in an IFN-γ dependent, TNF-α-independent manner.[62] As a result, immunological memory most likely does not carry over to the next transmission season. Unfortunately, natural infections do not seem to provoke the same memory CD4 T cell response afforded by low dose exposure to malaria. The vast array of malaria products known to modulate the host environment suggests that the parasite has likely developed mechanisms for manipulating the immune response to induce apoptosis of anti-malaria T cell populations.

---

[58] S. Crotty, R.J. Johnston and S.P. Schoenberger, Effectors and memories: Bcl-6 and Blimp-1 in T and B lymphocyte differentiation, *Nature Immunology,* **11**(2), 114–20.

[59] M.M. Stevenson *et al.*, IL-12-induced protection against blood-stage *Plasmodium chabaudi* AS requires IFN-Î³ and TNF-Î± and occurs via a nitric oxide-dependent mechanism, *Journal of Immunology*, 1995, **155**(5), 2545–56.

[60] G.E. Grau *et al.*, Tumor-necrosis factor and other cytokines in cerebral malaria: experimental and clinical data, *Immunological Reviews*, 1989, **112**, 49–70.

[61] D.J. Pombo *et al.*, Immunity to malaria after administration of ultra-low doses of red cells infected with *Plasmodium falciparum, Lancet*, 2002, **360**(9333), 610–7.

[62] H. Xu *et al.*, The mechanism and significance of deletion of parasite-specific CD4+ T cells in malaria infection, *Journal of Experimental Medicine*, 2002, **195**(7), 881–92.

CD4 T cells also contribute to parasite clearance by supporting other cell types. CD8 T cells undergo expansion and proliferation and increase their parasiticidal cytolytic activity in response to sporozoites antigens. However, in the absence of CD4 T cells, anti-malaria CD8 cells cannot be sustained past six days post infection. CD4 T cells may either support CD8 T cell survival or protect CD8 T cells from activation-induced cell death.[63] Since sporozoites and extraerythrocytic forms, the two parasite stages detectable to CD8 T cells, remain in the liver for 7–14 days post infection, CD4 T cell help is crucial for retaining an adequate cytolytic CD8 T cell response. Thus, despite the well-known anti-inflammatory functions of IL-4, this cytokine seems to be the major contributor to a sustained inflammatory CD8 response. IL-4 secreted by CD4 T cells also aids in the production of anti-malaria antibody. Activated CD4 T cells and B cells that recognize epitopes of the same antigen can interact via their antigen-bound MHC class II receptor and co-stimulatory molecules. During this interaction, the CD4 T cell promotes the activation of the B cell and its differentiation into antibody-secreting plasma cells by secreting IL-4 (and also to a lesser extent, IL-5 and IL-6). Infection of T and B cell deficient mice clearly demonstrate that CD4 T cells are required for full protection, even after reconstitution of B cells.[64] Malaria-specific CD4 T cells thus are central to both the acute and long term anti-malaria response, and the key to anti-malaria immunity may lie in the ability to properly harness the CD4 T cell response.

One major gap in the field of T cell biology and malaria infection is that most of the parasite peptides recognized by human and mouse CD4 T cells remain unknown. CD4 T cell receptors are specific for short epitopes of parasite peptides and identification of these epitopes will be greatly beneficial as a tool for isolation of malaria-specific T cell clones. Distinct malaria-specific T cell clones likely act differently in response to antigen recognition, and epitope recognition could allow for the detection of those clones that elicit a protective response. Stephens *et al.* successfully identified a P. chabaudi CD4 T cell epitope and they have generated a TCR transgenic mouse expressing this epitope.[64] Although this malaria CD4 TCR transgenic mouse has proven to be extraodinarily useful in studying CD4 T cell immunity, the extensive differences between the mouse and human parasite strains require that human CD4 T cell clones be identified and investigated. If a protective T cell clone is discovered, one can imagine designing a vaccine that specifically stimulates the proliferation and memory cell development of this specific clone.

[63]L.H. Carvalho *et al.*, IL-4-secreting CD4+ T cells are crucial to the development of CD8+ T-cell responses against malaria liver stages, *Nature Medicine*, 2002, **8**(2), 166–70.
[64]R. Stephens *et al.*, Malaria-specific transgenic CD4+ T cells protect immunodeficient mice from lethal infection and demonstrate requirement for a protective threshold of antibody production for parasite clearance, *Blood*, 2005, **106**(5), 1676–84.

CD8 T Cells

Early malaria immunologists made several seminal observations concerning CD8 T cells during malaria infection, which provided hope for the development of a protective vaccine. Since the 1980s, multiple laboratories have demonstrated that administration of gamma-irradiated malaria sporozoites via injection or mosquito bite can protect the host against subsequent infection to any of the mouse malaria species and to the human parasite *P. falciparum*.[65,66] Knowing that protective immunity is in fact achievable greatly encouraged the push for malaria vaccine development. In order to determine precisely which immune responses were protective for malaria infection, different immune components were analyzed in vaccinated mice to determine which were sufficient or required for protection.

In the 1980s, several groups showed that CD8 T cells and IFNγ were required for protective immunity while CD4 T cells and anti-malaria IgG antibodies contributed to a swift recall response but were dispensible for complete protection.[65,66] Since CD8 T cells are MHC class I restricted and thus cannot detect malaria parasites within red blood cells, the protective immune response elicited by vaccination with irradiated sporozoites most likely occurs at the sporozoite or liver stage. As research of parasite motility progressed concurrently with an improved understanding of host immune detection mechanisms, a picture of CD8 T cell priming and memory formation began to emerge. It appears that peripheral migratory dendritic cells encounter either sporozoites or parasite products near the site of the mosquito bite, in the lymphatics, or in circulation.[67] These dendritic cells then phagocytose the parasites or their products and migrate to a nearby draining lymph node. In these draining lymph nodes, the now mature dendritic cell presents malaria antigens to CD8 T cells, which activates the T cells to become effector T cells that home to the liver or spleen. In the liver, effector CD8 T cells induce killing of infected hepatocytes and control the infection.[68]

The mechanisms used by CD8 T cells to kill infected red blood cells have not been completely identified. IFN-γ, perforin, Fas and TNF-α-mediated cytotoxicity

[65]L. Schofield *et al.*, Gamma interferon, CD8+ T cells and antibodies required for immunity to malaria sporozoites, *Nature*, 1987, **330**(6149), 664–6.

[66]W.R. Weiss *et al.*, CD8+ T cells (cytotoxic/suppressors) are required for protection in mice immunized with malaria sporozoites, *Proceedings of the National Academy of Sciences of the United States of America*, 1988, **85**(2), 573–6.

[67]E. Segura and J.A. Villadangos, Antigen presentation by dendritic cells *in vivo*, *Current Opinions in Immunology*, 2009, **21**(1), 105–10.

[68]M.C. Seguin *et al.*, Induction of nitric oxide synthase protects against malaria in mice exposed to irradiated *Plasmodium berghei* infected mosquitoes: involvement of interferon gamma and CD8+ T cells, *Journal of Experimental Medicine*, 1994, **180**(1), 353–8.

have all been described, but no single mechanism has been identified to be essential for parasite killing. It is quite possible that some or any combinations of these mechanisms are sufficient to kill parasites and infected hepatocytes.[69]

A major hurdle in studying the CD8 response is that CD8 T cells appear to behave differently during malaria infection than during infections by most other pathogens. In general, CD8 T cells require CD4 T cell help during recall responses and not during primary infection. In malaria, CD8 T cells can confer protection after irradiated sporozoite immunization without CD4 T cell help; however, in order for CD8 T cells to sustain cytotoxicity during both primary and subsequent infections, CD4 T cells are required. More specifically, Carvalho *et al.* found that IL-4 secreted by CD4 T cells is necessary and sufficient for continued CD8 cytotoxicity after four days post infection. Considering that extraerythrocytic forms remain inside hepatocytes for about 1–2 weeks after *P. falciparum* infection, CD4 T cells likely play a major role in the initial immune response.

Another important difference between CD8 T cells in malaria infection and other pathogen infections is that CD8 T cells in malaria have more stringent requirements for priming by APCs. Upon infection, dendritic cells must initially prime CD8 T cells, but activation of the same T cell can only be accomplished by hepatocytes or other parenchymal cells that are not specialized antigen presenting cells.[70] Furthermore, malaria-specific CD8 T cell clones do not seem to undergo clonal expansion after prime-boost procedures as efficiently as CD8 T cell clones specific for other pathogens. 1–2 large doses of malaria antigen elicits more clonal expansion than multiple smaller doses.[71] It remains to be determined whether this phenomenon of CD8 clonal expansion aids or hinders vaccine development. On one hand, requiring only a single dose for protection would be ideal, but on the other hand, vaccines that rely on natural exposure for boosting may fail. These findings suggest that malaria-specific CD8 T cell expansion largely depends on the context in which the antigen is presented, and determining these criteria should be a main focus of vaccine development.

Regulatory T Cells

It has long been observed that the high levels of IFN-γ, TNF-α, IL-12 and other inflammatory cytokines expressed during the acute phase of malaria are

---

[69] D.L. Doolan and S.L. Hoffman, The complexity of protective immunity against liver-stage malaria, *Journal of Immunology*, 2000, **165**(3), 1453–62.

[70] S. Chakravarty *et al.*, CD8+ T lymphocytes protective against malaria liver stages are primed in skin-draining lymph nodes, *Nature Medicine*, 2007, **13**(9), 1035–41.

[71] J.C. Hafalla *et al.*, Short-term antigen presentation and single clonal burst limit the magnitude of the CD8(+) T cell responses to malaria liver stages, *Proceedings of the National Academy of Sciences of the United States of America*, 2002, **99**(18), 11819–24.

unsustainable and must be down-regulated to prevent excessive and often lethal end-organ damage.[11] However, reducing inflammation comes at the cost of permitting continued parasite growth. The temporal control of anti-inflammatory mediators must be tightly regulated so that pro-inflammatory responses dominate during the initial phase of infection to control parasite replication, and anti-inflammatory cytokines increase when parasite numbers have been substantially lowered or when continued inflammation would result in excessive host pathology or death.[72] At first, the anti-inflammatory mediators were thought to be induced by Th2 cells, but recent studies suggest that a different T cell subset, the regulatory T cell, is in fact mainly responsible for reducing the inflammatory response.[73]

Regulatory T cells dampen the host inflammatory response by secreting the anti-inflammatory cytokines IL-10 and TGF-β.[73] Details regarding the regulatory T cell response during malaria infection are controversial at best and largely unknown. The signals that activate regulatory T cells have not been identified, and the published roles of regulatory T cells vary depending on experimental design, malaria species, host species, and the timing of sample collection and analysis.[74] Furthermore, regulatory T cell genetic knockout mouse models do not currently exist and depletion of regulatory T cells by administration of neutralizing anti-CD25 antibodies is problematic,[75] leaving researchers with few practical options for directly studying the role of regulatory T cells in malaria.

The malaria regulatory T cell field generally agrees that the numbers of regulatory T cells increase during most mouse infection models;[76,77] however reports of both increased and decreased control of parasitemia and T cell proliferation as a result of regulatory T cell activation are found in the literature. In human studies, regulatory T cell changes are even more difficult to investigate. Since regulatory T cells are transiently upregulated and short-lived upon activation, the role of regulatory T cells is difficult to investigate in humans because one cannot determine when the infection occurred.

---

[72] F.M. Omer, J.A. Kurtzhals and E.M. Riley, Maintaining the immunological balance in parasitic infections: a role for TGF-beta?, *Parasitology Today*, 2000, **16**(1), 18–23.

[73] H. Groux *et al.*, A CD4+ T-cell subset inhibits antigen-specific T-cell responses and prevents colitis, *Nature*, 1997, **389**(6652), 737–42.

[74] O.C. Finney, E.M. Riley and M. Walther, Regulatory T cells in malaria–friend or foe?, *Trends in Immunology*, **31**(2), 63–70.

[75] K.N. Couper *et al.*, Incomplete depletion and rapid regeneration of Foxp3+ regulatory T cells following anti-CD25 treatment in malaria-infected mice, *Journal of Immunology*, 2007, **178**(7), 4136–46.

[76] M. Walther *et al.*, Upregulation of TGF-beta, FOXP3, and CD4+CD25+ regulatory T cells correlates with more rapid parasite growth in human malaria infection, *Immunity*, 2005, **23**(3), 287–96.

[77] H. Hisaeda *et al.*, Escape of malaria parasites from host immunity requires CD4+ CD25+ regulatory T cells, *Nature Medicine*, 2004, **10**(1), 29–30.

Stringent regulation of the anti-inflammatory response is of utmost importance because the appearance of regulatory T cells too early/too late or too many/too few can all result in host death from hyperparasitemia or immunopathology. Thus, a second layer of control exists at the level of cytokine activation: regulatory T cells produce TGF-β in a latent form which must then be activated to have anti-inflammatory properties.[78] An intriguing recent finding reports that *P. falciparum* and the laboratory rodent malaria species express proteins that can activate latent TGF-β.[79] This immunomodulatory mechanism may contribute significantly to diminished parasite clearance and should be considered when analyzing potent malaria effectors for treatment or vaccine targeting.

B Cells/Antibody

Many of the earliest treatments of severe malaria involve passive transfer of serum from 'immune' individuals,[80] and so antibodies have long been recognized as an important, if not essential, component of an effective anti-malaria response. As a blood-borne pathogen that is only exposed to the host for short periods of time prior to re-invasion, malaria parasites are a likely target for antibody responses. The importance of antibodies implies that the source of these antibodies — namely B cells and plasma cells — are also crucially involved in parasite clearance. Mice depleted of B cells cannot control an otherwise self-resolving infection with *P. chabaudi*, nor do they exhibit signs of immunological memory against a second infection (after treatment of the first infection). These defects however can be rescued by either passive transfer of immune serum or active transfer of immune B cells into the deficient mice.[81]

Our knowledge of the mechanism by which antibodies clear parasites remains incomplete. The host may employ many different mechanisms of antibody-mediated inhibition of parasites to combat the wide variety of parasite products that the host encounters during infection. One likely and perhaps dominant method by which antibodies eliminate parasites is via antibody activation of macrophages. The Fc region of antibodies can bind to mononuclear cells via the FcRγII surface

[78] J.L. Wrana *et al.*, Mechanism of activation of the TGF-beta receptor, *Nature*, 1994, **370**(6488), 341–7.

[79] F.M. Omer *et al.*, Activation of transforming growth factor beta by malaria parasite-derived metalloproteinases and a thrombospondin-like molecule, *Journal of Experimental Medicine*, 2003, **198**(12), 1817–27.

[80] S. Cohen, G.I. Mc and S. Carrington, Gamma-globulin and acquired immunity to human malaria, *Nature*, 1961, **192**, 733–7.

[81] T. von der Weid, N. Honarvar and J. Langhorne, Gene-targeted mice lacking B cells are unable to eliminate a blood stage malaria infection, *Journal of Immunology*, 1996, **156**(7), 2510–6.

receptor, and if antigens from the merozoites stage bind to these antibodies, they trigger activation of the monocytes to release soluble parasite inhibitors. Interestingly, this mechanism is specific for inhibiting only the nuclear division stage of the parasite life cycle, which makes it highly efficient at restricting infection once the parasites have reached the blood stage.[33]

Anti-malaria antibodies also can limit parasite growth at other life cycle stages. For example, sporozoites are susceptible to opsonizing antibodies as soon as these organisms enter the host.[82] The small number of sporozoites inoculated into the host should make anti-sporozoite antibodies highly effective; however, vaccine studies suggest that anti-sporozoite antibody retention and expansion is poor and cannot sustain protective immunity against subsequent infections. Invasion of the red blood cell is a highly coordinated event that involves both parasite and host surface antigens. Antibodies can prevent proteolytic processing of malaria invasion proteins as well as block the erythrocyte binding sites of malaria proteins, thereby hindering the invasion process and causing parasite death.[83] Anti-malaria antibodies also can recognize infected red blood cells by binding to malaria antigens that the parasite traffics to the surface of the cell. Once bound to the infected red blood cell, the antibodies induce the assembly of hemolytic complement which results in cell lysis.[84] Still other anti-malaria antibodies prevent rosetting and cytoadherence of infected red blood cells,[85] thus conferring protection from vessel occlusion and cerebral malaria while enhancing parasite recognition by immune cells.

Numerous population studies document increases in both overall antibody titers, especially IgG, and in malaria-specific antibody levels during and immediately following infection.[86,87] The spike in overall antibody levels likely results from the wide array of malaria antigens present in the host and most of these are

---

[82] H. Groux and J. Gysin, Opsonization as an effector mechanism in human protection against asexual blood stages of *Plasmodium falciparum*: Functional role of IgG subclasses, *Research in Immunology*, 1990, **141**(6), 529–42.

[83] M.J. Blackman *et al.*, Antibodies inhibit the protease-mediated processing of a malaria merozoite surface protein, *Journal of Experimental Medicine*, 1994, **180**(1), 389–93.

[84] J. Healer *et al.*, Complement-mediated lysis of *Plasmodium falciparum* gametes by malaria-immune human sera is associated with antibodies to the gamete surface antigen Pfs230, *Infection and Immunity*, 1997, **65**(8), 3017–23.

[85] J. Carlson *et al.*, Human cerebral malaria: association with erythrocyte rosetting and lack of anti-rosetting antibodies, *Lancet*, 1990, **336**(8729), 1457–60.

[86] I.A. McGregor *et al.*, Plasma immunoglobulin concentrations in an African (Gambian) community in relation to season, malaria and other infections and pregnancy, *Clinical and Experimental Immunology*, 1970, **7**(1), 51–74.

[87] J.E. Tobie *et al.*, Serum immunoglobulin levels in human malaria and their relationship to antibody production, *Journal of Immunology*, 1966, **97**(4), 498–505.

actually cross-reactive rather than malaria-specific antibodies. Not only are cross-reactive antibodies unable to sustain a protective anti-malaria response, but overwhelming levels of non-specific antibodies may actually impede the function of pathogen-specific antibodies.[88] Weiss *et al.* recently published evidence supporting slow development of immunity, as opposed to destruction of established immunity, by tracking development and persistence of malaria antibodies from the malarious wet season through the non-malarious dry season to the next malaria season. They compared both malaria specific and non-specific antibodies with anti-tetanus antibodies, which are known to confer long term protection after a single vaccination, and found that unlike the response to tetanus, malaria-specific antibodies are very slow to develop. Anti-malaria antibodies peak at the end of the malaria season, but rapidly decline during the dry season so that at the beginning of the next wet season, anti-malaria antibody titers are only slightly higher than titers at the start of the previous wet season. In this way, anti-malaria antibodies accumulate extremely slowly[89] and this may explain why protection takes years to develop and can be rapidly lost.

Anti-malaria antibody responses, or lack thereof, should be analyzed in the context of B cell and plasma cell responses during malaria infection as these cells are responsible for the production of antibody. During infection, most of the antigen presentation interactions occur in the spleen. B cells with B cell receptors bound to malaria antigens require a second signal for full activation. The antigen-bound B cells migrate to the T cell zones, and are activated upon encounter with helper T cells presenting both an associated malaria antigen and co-stimulatory ligands. Once activated, the B cell disengages from the helper T cell and either proliferates to form germinal centers or migrates to the red pulp. Activated B cells in the red pulp undergo clonal expansion and eventually become long and short-lived plasma cells that secret antigen. Short-lived plasma cells are cleared quickly following infection, and long-lived plasma cells travel to the bone marrow, probably requiring frequent antigen stimulation to be sustained. Germinal center B cells undergo somatic hypermutation to generate B cell receptors (BCRs) with extremely high affinity for malaria antigens. B cells with highly specific B cell receptors then become either memory B cells or plasma cells.[90] The process of somatic hypermutation also depends on the pres-

---

[88]J.A. Guevara Patino *et al.*, Antibodies that inhibit malaria merozoite surface protein-1 processing and erythrocyte invasion are blocked by naturally acquired human antibodies, *Journal of Experimental Medicine*, 1997, **186**(10), 1689–99.

[89]G.E. Weiss *et al.*, The *Plasmodium falciparum*-specific human memory B cell compartment expands gradually with repeated malaria infections, *Public Library of Science Pathogens*, **6**(5), e1000912.

[90]S.K. Pierce, Understanding B cell activation: from single molecule tracking, through Tolls, to stalking memory in malaria, *Immunologic Research*, 2009, **43**(1–3), 85–97.

ence of malaria antigens, thus the availability of malaria antigens and the context in which the antigens are presented could present a bottleneck for the acquisition of sterile humoral immunity. Wykes *et al.* also reported that malaria infection induces apoptosis of malaria-specific B cells generated by immunization, further hindering the humoral anti-malaria response.[91]

Coping with Malaria — Tolerance, Immune Evasion, Genetic Polymorphisms

In a two-year longitudinal study in Gabon, Lell *et al.* found that children who presented at the hospital with symptoms of severe malaria had significantly greater chances of reinfection during subsequent transmission seasons. Even more unfortunate for these children, their symptoms during future infections continued to be more severe than the disease symptoms of those who presented initially with mild malaria.[92] With all other assessable factors — mosquito inoculation rate, socioeconomic class, access to hospitals — being equal, these findings suggest that host genetic polymorphisms dictate malaria disease severity. Indeed, when taken together with the knowledge that *P. falciparum* is estimated to have evolved with the human population for the past 2.5 million years,[93] malaria certainly exerted evolutionary pressures that shaped the human genome.

Association studies have demonstrated that polymorphisms in numerous genes are linked to susceptibility of malaria infection and disease severity. These polymorphisms are found in three general classes of genes: red blood cell protein, antigen presentation and cytokine signaling, and adhesion molecule expression. Polymorphisms in red blood cell protein-related genes offer some of the most well known examples of the selective pressure exerted by malaria. Red blood cell polymorphisms like the hemoglobin S (HbS) sickle cell trait[94] and α- and β-thalassemias[95] are often pathologic or fatal in the homozygous recessive form, but are retained at extraordinarily high rates within certain genetic pools because of the protection conferred to heterozygous individuals. Other red blood cell polymorphisms that affect malaria infection are the hemoglobin C (HbC) trait,[94] glucose-6-phosphate

---

[91] M.N. Wykes *et al.*, *Plasmodium yoelii* can ablate vaccine-induced long-term protection in mice, *Journal of Immunology*, 2005, **175**(4), 2510–6.

[92] B. Lell *et al.*, The role of red blood cell polymorphisms in resistance and susceptibility to malaria, *Clinical Infectious Diseases*, 1999, **28**(4), 794–9.

[93] R.E. Ricklefs and D.C. Outlaw, A molecular clock for malaria parasites, *Science*. 329(5988), 226–9.

[94] F. Verra *et al.*, Haemoglobin C and S role in acquired immunity against *Plasmodium falciparum* malaria, *Public Library of Science One*, 2007, **2**(10), e978.

[95] R. Udomsangpetch *et al.*, Alteration in cytoadherence and rosetting of *Plasmodium falciparum*-infected thalassemic red blood cells, *Blood*, 1993, **82**(12), 3752–9.

deficiency (G6PD),[96] and the Duffy antigen null trait.[97] The main source of nutrients for malaria parasites is hemoglobin from the host red blood cell, and it is likely that many of the above genetic polymorphisms result in an altered Hb structure that is poorly metabolized by the plasmodium parasite. *P. vivax* must bind to the Duffy antigen on the red blood cell surface in order to invade the red blood cell; thus individuals who lack the Duffy antigen are protected from *P. vivax* infection.[97] Superimposed maps of these genetic polymorphisms with areas of high malaria transmission are highly congruous and strongly suggest that humans have adapted to living with the malaria parasite.

The next two classes of genetic polymorphisms affect mostly disease outcome or severity rather than susceptibility. As discussed in previous sections, the ability to regulate the inflammatory response to malaria infection affects not only disease severity and outcome, but also generation of memory responses. It is not surprising then that numerous polymorphisms are found in promoter regions that regulate cytokine expression. For example, an IL-12 promoter polymorphism has been associated with decreased incidence of cerebral malaria. As discussed previously, increased levels of IL-12 activates IFN-γ-secreting T cells, which then activate monocytes to induce NO and kill parasites.[98] Individuals homozygous for the IL-12Bpro2 gene produce more bioactive IL-12 upon ligation of co-stimulatory molecules and are protected from cerebral malaria.[98,99] Another example of a genetic polymorphism adapted to malaria is found in the promoter region of the macrophage migration inhibitory factor (MIF) gene. MIF is a cytokine that can orchestrate a potent inflammatory response through its ability to inhibit activation induced apoptosis of macrophages and promote expression of other inflammatory cytokines such as IL-6 and TNF-α. MIF expression is regulated by a microsatellite repeat in the 5' untranslated region that regulates levels of MIF secretion upon infection. High levels of MIF expression are detrimental for surviving malaria infection and causes increased anemia.[100]

[96] S.A. Tishkoff *et al.*, Haplotype diversity and linkage disequilibrium at human G6PD: recent origin of alleles that confer malarial resistance, *Science*, 2001, **293**(5529), 455–62.

[97] L.H. Miller*et al.*, The resistance factor to *Plasmodium vivax* in blacks. The Duffy-blood-group genotype, FyFy, *New England Journal of Medicine*, 1976, **295**(6), 302–4.

[98] G. Morahan *et al.*, A promoter polymorphism in the gene encoding interleukin-12 p40 (IL12B) is associated with mortality from cerebral malaria and with reduced nitric oxide production, *Genes and Immunity*, 2002, **3**(7), 414–8.

[99] J. Muller-Berghaus *et al.*, Deficient IL-12p70 secretion by dendritic cells based on IL12B promoter genotype, *Genes and Immunity*, 2004, **5**(5), 431–4.

[100] M.A. McDevitt *et al.*, A critical role for the host mediator macrophage migration inhibitory factor in the pathogenesis of malarial anemia, *Journal of Experimental Medicine*, 2006, **203**(5), 1185–96.

Interestingly, the highest frequency of low MIF-expressing alleles is found in the malarious regions of the world, suggesting another human adaptation to the parasite.[101,102]

During the red blood cell stages, malaria parasites attach to endothelial cells that line blood vessels to sequester it from sentinel immune cells. The parasites bind to the endothelium via adhesion molecules, which are upregulated during the innate inflammatory response to malaria infection. Sequestration of parasite prevents the spleen from clearing the infection, and humans have evolved polymorphisms in several adhesion molecule genes to subvert sequestration. One example of a host polymorphism is in ICAM-1. A mutation in ICAM-1 that affects malaria parasite binding was found in increased frequencies in several populations susceptible to malaria.[103] Although the protective effects of this mutation are still under investigation, it is likely the result of human co-evolution with malaria. Adhesion molecules like ICAM-1 are upregulated during the innate inflammatory response to malaria blood stage infection, and the parasites.[104] Numerous other genetic polymorphisms have been associated with malaria disease severity, including inflammatory factors MHC,[105] TNF-α,[106] regulatory T cell frequencies[107] and adhesion proteins CD36[108] and CD31.[109]

---

[101] X.B. Zhong *et al.*, Simultaneous detection of microsatellite repeats and SNPs in the macrophage migration inhibitory factor (MIF) gene by thin-film biosensor chips and application to rural field studies, *Nucleic Acids Research*, 2005, **33**(13), e121.

[102] G.A. Awandare *et al.*, MIF (macrophage migration inhibitory factor) promoter polymorphisms and susceptibility to severe malarial anemia, *Journal of Infectious Diseases*, 2009, **200**(4), 629–37.

[103] D. Fernandez-Reyes *et al.*, A high frequency African coding polymorphism in the N-terminal domain of ICAM-1 predisposing to cerebral malaria in Kenya, *Human Molecular Genetics*, 1997, **6**(8), 1357–60.

[104] S.J. Chakravorty and A. Craig, The role of ICAM-1 in *Plasmodium falciparum* cytoadherence, *European Journal of Cell Biology*, 2005, **84**(1), 15–27.

[105] A. Jepson *et al.*, Genetic linkage of mild malaria to the major histocompatibility complex in Gambian children: study of affected sibling pairs, *British Medical Journal*, 1997, **315**(7100), 96–7.

[106] J.C. Knight *et al.*, A polymorphism that affects OCT-1 binding to the TNF promoter region is associated with severe malaria, *Nature Genetics*, 1999, **22**(2), 145–50.

[107] M.G. Torcia *et al.*, Functional deficit of T regulatory cells in Fulani, an ethnic group with low susceptibility to *Plasmodium falciparum* malaria, *Proceedings of the National Academy of Sciences of the United States of America*, 2008, **105**(2), 646–51.

[108] A. Pain *et al.*, A non-sense mutation in Cd36 gene is associated with protection from severe malaria, *Lancet*, 2001, **357**(9267), 1502–3.

[109] M. Kikuchi *et al.*, Association of adhesion molecule PECAM-1/CD31 polymorphism with susceptibility to cerebral malaria in Thais, *Parasitology International*, 2001, **50**(4), 235–9.

A distinct strategy of human adaptation to malaria infection is to tolerate the presence of parasites by limiting pathology rather than to eliminate the infection. Expression of heme oxygenase is a rare example of pathogen tolerance in humans.[110] An increase in TNF-α during malaria infection causes the release of free heme. Free heme is extremely cytotoxic and contributes to liver failure by inducing apoptosis of hepatocytes. Heme oxygenase is an enzyme that is involved in the degradation of free heme into non-toxic substrates, and thus expression of heme oxygenase during malaria protects the host from lethal liver damage without interfering with parasite burden.[111] Although malaria parasites constantly evolve to circumvent the host immune response, millions of years of co-evolution have allowed the human host to find numerous ways of adapting to malaria infection.

Conclusion

The full picture of an optimal immune response to malaria is not yet clear, but pieces of the puzzle are continuously being added. We now understand that anti-malaria antibodies and CD4 and CD8 memory T cells can all be generated after infection, and that regulated increases in IL-12 and IFN-γ are crucial for an adequate immune response. This knowledge is encouraging because it demonstrates that immunity can be achieved, but the problem that remains is how to simultaneously induce and regulate these responses so that a clinically significant protective response can be achieved.

Malaria is one of the oldest pathogens of humans, and the diversity of mechanisms that humans have evolved to survive malaria infections is somewhat astounding. Some of these mechanisms could potentially be channeled into the development of a vaccine;[112] however, this very genetic diversity poses another challenge for vaccine development. Disrupting the balance between the human host and malaria will likely have unpredictable and widely varying effects in different populations, some of which may be detrimental. Moreover, malaria parasites have co-evolved numerous ways of subverting the human immune system. Different isolates of the same malaria species rely on different mechanisms of

---

[110]R. Medzhitov, Damage control in host-pathogen interactions. *Proceedings of the National Academy of Sciences of the United States of America*, 2009, **106**(37), 15525–6.

[111]E. Seixas *et al.*, Heme oxygenase-1 affords protection against noncerebral forms of severe malaria, *Proceedings of the National Academy of Sciences of the United States of America*, 2009, **106**(37), 15837–42.

[112]S.K. Pierce and L.H. Miller, World Malaria Day 2009: what malaria knows about the immune system that immunologists still do not, *Journal of Immunology*, 2009, **182**(9), 5171–7.

invasion and evasion, so an effective vaccine will likely have to block several fundamental parasite processes.

Much is at stake for the development of a malaria vaccine to control malaria. Based on the current state of malaria research, a protective vaccine is plausible, but the many gaps in our understanding of the parasite biology and the host immune response continue to delay vaccine development.

Index

Printed in the United States
By Bookmasters